Management of Acute Coronary Syndromes

EDITED BY

PETER M SCHOFIELD MD, FRCP, FICA, FACC, FESC

CONSULTANT CARDIOLOGIST

CARDIAC UNIT

PAPWORTH HOSPITAL

PAPWORTH EVERARD

CAMBRIDGE

UK

MARTIN DUNITZ

© Martin Dunitz 2000

First published in the United Kingdom in 2000 by:
Martin Dunitz Ltd
The Livery House
7–9 Pratt Street
London NW1 0AE

Tel: +44 (0)207 482 2202
Fax: +44 (0)207 267 0159
E-mail: info@mdunitz.globalnet.co.uk
Website: http://www.dunitz.co.uk

A CIP record for this book is available from the British Library

ISBN 1-85317-719-9

Distributed in the United States by:
Blackwell Science Inc
Commerce Place, 350 Main Street
Malden MA 02148, USA
Tel: 1 800 215 1000

Distributed in Canada by:
Login Brothers Book Company
324 Salteaux Crescent
Winnipeg, Manitoba R3J 3T2
Canada
Tel: 1 204 224 4068

Distributed in Brazil by:
Ernesto Reichmann Distribuidora de Livros, Ltda
Rua Coronel Marques 335, Tatuape 03440-000
Sao Paulo
Brazil

Composition by Wearset, Boldon, Tyne and Wear
Printed and bound in Italy by Printer Trento

Contents

II Myocardial Infarction

Contributors

Inderpaul Birdi BMedSci(Hon), BM, BS, FRCS(Eng), MCh(Bristol)
Department of Cardiology, Cardiac Unit, Papworth Hospital,
Papworth Everard, Cambridge CB3 8RE

Adrian Brodison MB ChB, MRCP
Specialist Registrar in Cardiology, Regional Cardiothoracic
Centre, Blackpool Victoria Hospital, Blackpool FY3 8NR

Maurice B Buchalter MD
Consultant Cardiologist, Department of Cardiology,
University Hospital of Wales, Heath Park, Cardiff CF4 4XW

Michael H Cave MD, FRCP
Consultant Physician and Cardiologist, Dryburn Hospital,
Durham D11 5TW

Anoop Chauhan MD, MRCP
Consultant Cardiologist, Regional Cardiothoracic Centre,
Blackpool Victoria Hospital, Blackpool FY3 8NR

Andrew A Grace MB, PhD, MRCP, FACC
BHF Senior Research Fellow, Department of Biochemistry,
University of Cambridge, Cambridge CB2 1QW

James A Hall MA, MD, FRCP
Consultant Cardiologist, Cardiothoracic Unit,
South Cleveland Hospital, Middlesbrough,
Cleveland TS4 3BW

Antoinette Kenny MD, FRCP, FRCPI
Consultant Cardiologist, Freeman Hospital,
High Heaton, Newcastle upon Tyne NE7
7DN

Stephen R Large FRCS
Consultant Cardiothoracic Surgeon,
Department of Cardiology, Cardiac Unit,
Papworth Hospital, Papworth Everard,
Cambridge CB3 8RE

Peter F Ludman MA, MD, MRCP, FESC
Consultant Cardiologist, Birmingham
Heartlands and Solihull NHS Trust,
Birmingham Heartlands Hospital,
Birmingham B9 5SS

Paul A Mullins MD, FRCP
Consultant Physician and Cardiologist,
Royal Liverpool University Hospitals,
Liverpool L7 8XP

Kim Priestley MB, ChB, FRCP
Consultant Cardiologist, Birmingham
Heartlands and Solihull NHS Trust, Solihull
Hospital, Solihull, B91 2JL

Jason Pyatt MRCP
Specialist Registrar in Cardiology, The
Cardiothoracic Centre – Liverpool, NHS
Trust, Liverpool L14 3PE

Adrian D Raybould MD
Department of Cardiology, University
Hospital of Wales, Heath Park, Cardiff CF4
4XW

Andrew J Ritchie FRCS
Consultant Cardiothoracic Surgeon,
Department of Cardiology, Papworth
Hospital, Papworth Everard, Cambridge CB3
8RE

Rosemary A Rusk MB, MRCP
Specialist Registrar in Cardiology, Freeman
Hospital, High Heaton, Newcastle upon Tyne
NE7 7DN

Rana A Sayeed MRCP, FRCS
Medical Research Council Clinical Training
Fellow, Department of Biochemistry,
University of Cambridge, Cambridge CB2
1QW

Trevor Wistow MB BS (Hons), BSc, MRCP
Consultant Cardiologist, Department of
Cardiology, Norfolk & Norwich Healthcare
Trust, Norwich NR1 3SR

Foreword

Unstable coronary syndromes are medical emergencies. An atheromatous plaque in a major coronary artery has ulcerated, platelets are aggregating on the now exposed, raw, lipid-rich, inflamed plaque core and strands of fibrin are wafting in the arterial blood. More platelets accumulate and threaten to block the artery; some break off downstream. The clinical consequences of this include myocardial death and ventricular fibrillation.

The onset of unstable angina and myocardial infarction can be very difficult to diagnose. Even the most experienced patients, those who have suffered cardiac pain before, often fail to recognize the recurrence. Delay in presentation is, therefore, commonplace. On admission, there may be no abnormal signs and the initial electrocardiogram and early blood tests may also be normal. What should the clinician do? Some patients will continue to experience pain and undergo angiography with normal findings. These and many others will have non-cardiac diagnoses – chest wall pain for example. Other scenarios include patients whose unstable coronary syndromes have been recognized and appropriately treated but who suffer further episodes of pain and infarction, which are only recognized belatedly because they have been transferred to a low-intensity care area; or the patients whose stuttering myocardial infarcts progress inexorably despite expert cardiological intervention.

Few countries can afford the luxury of coronary angiography for all those patients with unstable coronary syndromes, with revascularization for some, yet this might be the right approach. Coronary intervention is certainly exciting and dramatic, but for whom? Most patients in UK practice are elderly, have other pathologies and three-vessel coronary disease; and they may have to wait endlessly for coronary bypass surgery. Treatment is therefore compromised by lack of resources. Moreover, those patients recruited to clinical trials seldom seem to resemble those facing us in the coronary care unit, and when we come to consider modern drug treatment, notably the platelet glycoprotein IIb/IIIa inhibitors, we again face

the issue of cost. And are we sure that we are using the tried and tested drugs to maximum effect?

The 'evidence base' for the management of patients with unstable coronary syndromes may thus be absent or inapplicable. There is an urgent need for books such as this one which bring together the skills and experience of clinicians who face these problems daily. The authors have complementary talents and many have made unique contributions to the cardiology service in Cambridge. The ideas and management policies synthesized in this book are an admirable blend of theory and practice, taking into account the results of published data. The result is a welcome addition to the cardiological literature.

Michael C Petch MD, FRCP, FACC, FESC
Consultant Cardiologist
Papworth Hospital
Cambridge

I Unstable Angina

History, examination and investigations (including pathophysiology and epidemiology)

Trevor Wistow

1

Introduction

Unstable angina is one of the commonest cardiac diagnoses resulting in admission to the coronary care unit or cardiac ward. In 1991, the US National Center for Health Statistics reported 570 000 hospital admissions with a diagnosis of unstable angina, resulting in 3.1 million hospital days.[1]

Over the last decade or so, advances in the understanding of the pathogenesis of unstable angina have been translated into therapeutic benefit. Standard care of these patients now involves treatment with aspirin,[2] heparin,[3] beta-blockers[4] and nitrates. Interventional cardiologists have had an increasing role to play, particularly with the advent of coronary stents. More recently, evidence has emerged supporting the use of other inhibitors of platelet aggregation, particularly the glycoprotein IIa/IIIb inhibitors[5,6] either as an adjunct to interventional techniques or on the coronary care unit.

It is therefore essential that the physician caring for patients with unstable angina has a thorough understanding of the underlying pathophysiological processes, together with the ability to select those patients at high risk who may benefit from more aggressive management.

Definition of unstable angina

Crescendo angina, pre-infarction angina and the intermediate syndrome are a few of the terms previously used to describe the syndrome we now call unstable angina. The variety of names reflects the heterogeneous nature of the condition both in terms of clinical presentation and outcome. This label of unstable angina does however serve a useful purpose in identifying a population of patients with coronary disease sharing a common pathophysiology, who warrant more intensive investigation and treatment.

Most definitions recognize three presentations:[7]

- Angina at rest of a prolonged nature (>20 minutes).
- Recent onset severe angina (at least Canadian Cardiovascular Score III).
- Recent acceleration of angina to at least Canadian Cardiovascular Score III.

These definitions require the exclusion of myocardial infarction (MI). Although conventional cardiac enzymes (CK_{MB}, AST, LDH) are not elevated, troponin T or I are frequently detected indicating that minor

degrees of myocardial damage do occur (see below).

Post-MI angina and non-Q-wave MI are part of the same clinical spectrum. Although variant (or Prinzmetal's) angina causes recurrent attacks of rest angina, it is not considered here as the pathophysiology is different.[8]

Braunwald has proposed a classification of unstable angina focusing on the severity of symptoms, the clinical circumstances in which unstable angina occurs and whether there are electrocardiographic (ECG) changes during episodes of chest pain.[9]

The severity of symptoms is classed I–III. Class I is new onset severe or accelerated angina. Class II refers to those with rest pain over the last month but not preceding 48 h. Class III identifies patients with one or more episodes of rest pain within the preceding 48 hours. The clinical circumstances in which angina occurred is assigned A, B or C. In Class A or secondary unstable angina there is a clear precipitating cause, e.g. anaemia. Class B angina describes those in whom unstable angina develops without an extra cardiac precipitant. Class C is post-infarction unstable angina. The presence or absence of transient ST and T abnormalities is also noted. Prospective trials have demonstrated that the classification is helpful in predicting those patients with a poor outlook and who are likely to require intervention.[10,11]

Pathophysiology

All myocardial ischaemia results from an imbalance between myocardial oxygen demand and supply, most commonly due to severe disease in one or more of the coronary vessels.[12] In chronic stable angina pectoris, ischaemia is the result of stenosed arteries being unable to deliver sufficient blood supply at times of increased demand such as exercise or emotional stress. By contrast, in unstable angina, the major cause of this imbalance is a reduction in supply. This primary reduction in supply has been demonstrated in haemodynamic and ECG studies, where ischaemic ECG changes and reversible (ischaemic) left ventricular dysfunction occur independently of factors that increase myocardial oxygen demands, such as heart rate or arterial blood pressure.[13,14]

In most cases of unstable angina we now know the cause of the reduction in myocardial blood supply to be a non-occlusive, labile thrombus superimposed on a fissured or eroded atheromatous plaque.[15] Transient episodes of thrombotic occlusion may occur and local vasoconstriction further reduces coronary blood flow.[16] In some cases, however, progressive and rapid severe mechanical obstruction due to plaque expansion is undoubtedly important.[17]

Patients with hitherto stable coronary artery disease may develop unstable symptoms due to secondary factors that may precipitate an unstable episode. Examples of this include febrile illness, anaemia, thyrotoxicosis, hypoxia, uncontrolled hypertension, hypotension arrhythmias and the withdrawal of antianginal therapy, particularly beta-blockers.[9]

Plaque rupture

There appears to be little relationship between the severity of stenosis of a plaque and its vulnerability to rupture.[18] Many episodes of unstable angina or MI occur in vessels that are only mild or moderately stenotic. The morphology of the plaque and extrinsic factors appear to be more important.

Those atheromatous plaques that are most likely to rupture are eccentric with a thin, fibrous cap and decreased amount of collagen between the lumen and a large lipid pool.[19] The site of rupture is often the junction between the eccentric plaque and the normal vessel wall, where shear forces are prominent. Fluctuations in arterial pressure may play a role.[18] The content of the plaque is highly thrombogenic. Both the lipid pool and subendothelial collagen, when exposed to the blood stream, activate platelets and promote thrombus formation.[18]

Thrombosis and platelet aggregation

Platelet aggregation and thrombus formation are key elements in the pathogenesis of unstable angina. Filling defects suggestive of thrombus are frequently seen in angiograms of patients with unstable angina[20] and angioscopic studies suggest that thrombus is present in virtually all cases.[21] The findings differ, however, from those found in acute MI. In unstable angina, thrombus often has a greyish appearance suggesting that the clot mainly consists of platelets, whereas in MI the clot is red suggesting a predominance of erythrocytes.[21] Post-mortem studies in patients who die suddenly with unstable angina confirm the presence of thrombus in most cases; moreover platelet emboli are often evident within intramyocardial small vessels.[22]

Metabolites of thromboxane A_2 derived from platelets are found in increased concentrations in the urine of some patients with unstable angina.[23] This, together with serum markers of thrombin generation and fibrin formation (fibrinopeptide A, prothrombin I and II, D-dimer),[24,25] provide indirect evidence of the importance of thrombosis and platelet aggregation.

Clinical trials pointing to the benefits of anti-aggregatory drugs such as aspirin,[2] ticlopidine[26] and the glycoprotein IIIa/IIb inhibitors[5,6] in the management of unstable coronary disease underline the importance of platelet activation and thrombosis in the pathogenesis.

Vasoconstriction

Vasoconstriction plays an important role in unstable angina.[16] It is thought that both endothelial dysfunction and vasoactive compounds produced by platelets contribute to abnormal vasomotor tone.

Healthy endothelium synthesizes nitric oxide, prostacyclin and tissue plasminogen activator (TPA) which inhibit vasoconstriction and platelet aggregation. Loss of normal endothelium results in reduced local concentrations of these compounds and a vasoconstrictive response to the vasodilatory compounds acetylcholine, bradykinin and serotonin.[27] It is possible that disrupted endothelium leads to local increases in the vasoconstrictor endothelin.[28]

Aggregating platelets synthesize and release serotonin and thromboxane A_2, which is a potent vasoconstrictor.[27] Thrombin may also directly act on damaged endothelium causing vasoconstriction.

The role of inflammation

Although plaque fissuring and thrombus formation underlie most cases of unstable angina, autopsy studies show no erosion of fissuring in a significant minority.[29] It is possible that an inflammatory process may contribute to thrombosis and vasoconstriction. Inflammatory cells present at the shoulder of atheromatous plaques, producing cytokines which may interact with endothelium to promote thrombosis and vasoconstriction. Inflammation probably plays an important part in plaque rupture. Macrophages and T lymphocytes are able to degrade the plaque by the secretion of proteolytic enzymes.[30]

Clinical studies have supported the concept that inflammation may be important in the acute coronary syndromes as there appears to be an association with the acute phase reactants C-reactive protein and amyloid A protein with adverse clinical outcomes.[31,32] The trigger for an inflammatory process is unknown, though there has been much speculation about the possibility of an infectious agent. Serology of patients with acute coronary syndromes show that infection with *Chlamydia pneumoniae, Helicobacter pylori* and cytomegalovirus are common.[33] Whether these have a causative role is unknown,[34] however small clinical trials using macrolide antibiotics have suggested possible benefits in patients with acute coronary syndromes, lending support to the theory that infectious agents may be important.[35]

Common pathogenesis of unstable coronary syndromes

Plaque rupture occurs in stable and unstable coronary disease. In stable coronary disease it is more limited, and thrombus does not extend into the lumen. Plaque ruptures that expose large areas of thrombogenic intramural debris to flowing blood in areas of high turbulence are most likely to provoke thrombosis within the lumen resulting in the unstable coronary syndromes.[18]

We now believe that unstable angina, non-Q-wave MI and Q-wave MI share a common pathogenesis. All three conditions result from plaque rupture leading to thrombosis, but in unstable angina the degree of plaque rupture may not be too extensive. Thrombotic occlusion is transient and vasoconstriction is prominent. More extensive plaque damage and longer thrombotic occlusion may lead to non-Q-wave MI; Q-wave MI results from complete and more persistent thrombotic occlusion. All three conditions are therefore part of a continuum. The extent of plaque disruption, exogenous thrombotic factors, vasoconstriction, presence of collateral circulation and spontaneous clot lysis are all factors that influence the clinical expression of plaque disruption.[36]

Clinical features

History

Patients typically present with chest discomfort, which although of a similar quality to stable angina, is often more severe and takes a different pattern. The amount of activity needed to reproduce symptoms may be minimal and patients may report an abrupt deterioration in exercise tolerance. For patients with previously stable disease they may notice that rest no longer relieves symptoms and that sublingual nitrate is less helpful or ineffective. Angina is typically prolonged perhaps lasting 20–30 min. Rest angina is a key feature. Some report additional features such as sweating, nausea or dizziness together with pain.

Some individuals with severe stable angina may experience very variable symptoms including nocturnal angina. A deterioration in their normal pattern is more important here than the exact circumstances in which angina occurs.

For patients with a new presentation of unstable angina it is vital to enquire about coronary risk factors and evidence of other vascular disease. Individuals with no risk factors, atypical features and a normal ECG form a low risk group for coronary events.

Examination

There are no specific physical signs that identify unstable angina. Some patients are pale and sweaty when in pain and there may be a tachycardia. Clinical evidence of impaired left ventricular function such as a gallop rhythm or basal crackles point to an individual at high risk. Hypotension is an ominous feature and transient mitral regurgitation is also associated with a poor outlook.

Investigations in unstable angina

The electrocardiogram

The electrocardiogram (ECG) gives invaluable information in the patient with unstable angina. Transient ST segment changes provide confirmatory evidence for a suspected diagnosis. Minor T wave changes are commonly seen but are less sensitive or specific for myocardial ischaemia.[37] Many patients have normal ECGs on presentation and although this does not exclude the diagnosis of unstable angina, it generally points to a favourable prognosis. Persistent ST segment depression (>12 h) usually suggests a diagnosis of non-Q-wave MI.

Changes on the ECG can also identify high-risk patients. Dynamic ST segment depression, occurring with pain which partially or completely resolves, indicates a group with a significant incidence of subsequent MI and death.[38,39] The magnitude of ST segment depression (in mm) is also significantly related to adverse outcome; generally speaking, the deeper the ST depression the worse the prognosis.[40] Extensive ECG changes on admission, i.e. both anterior and inferior ST depression, are strongly associated with triple vessel disease and left main stream stenosis. Unfortunately, ECG changes in patients with left main stem disease and unstable angina are neither sensitive or specific enough to enable the clinician to consistently predict anatomical findings based on the ECG.[41]

There are other ECG appearances which suggest an individual is at high risk. For example, deep, symmetrical T wave inversion in the anteroseptal leads is strongly associated with high-grade stenosis in the left anterior descending artery.[42,43] This population benefits from an aggressive approach with early revascularization. Patients with left bundle branch block or ECG evidence of previous MI are likely to have impaired left ventricular function with or without multivessel coronary disease, which are both pointers to a worse outcome.[37]

Continuous ST segment monitoring

Patients with stable coronary disease are known to have episodes of asymptomatic myocardial ischaemia, a phenomenon known as silent ischaemia. Continuous ST segment monitoring shows that in patients with unstable angina, frequent transient periods of ST depression also occur in the absence of symptoms. Some studies have suggested that the presence of ST depression or Holter monitoring is an independent predictor of adverse outcome.[44,45] This technique is not currently used routinely in the management of patients with unstable coronary syndromes, but it confirms that ongoing ischaemia, whether silent or symptomatic, indicates a risk of future coronary events.

Exercise testing

Patients who settle with medical therapy and who do not have features indicating high risk may undergo exercise ECG prior to discharge. In an individual with no ongoing symptoms and a normal ECG, a negative treadmill test points to an excellent prognosis.[46] Those patients with a positive exercise test, particularly those who are unable to manage four METS, and who have deep, widespread or prolonged ST depression, have a high incidence of future cardiac events and should be strongly considered for angiography with a view to revascularization.

Nuclear cardiology

Myocardial perfusion scanning is a very useful alternative to exercise ECG in assessing the need for more invasive investigation. High-risk features with thalium (Tl) scanning include perfusion defects in different territories indicating multivessel disease and increased lung uptake of Tl, which reflects exercise-induced left ventricular dysfunction.[47]

Echocardiography

The echocardiogram does not provide direct diagnostic findings in unstable angina but it may be useful in the risk stratification of patients. The presence of impaired left ventricular function (ejection fraction <40%), significant mitral regurgitation or regional wall abnormalities have all been found to point to an adverse prognosis.[48] Stress echocardiography provides additional prognostic information in those patients whose unstable symptoms have settled.

Laboratory investigations

Routine laboratory investigations usually show no specific abnormalities. The haemoglobin should always be measured to exclude anaemia. The white cell count is normally not elevated, in contrast to those patients with MI. Cardiac enzymes by definition are not elevated. A lipid profile should be arranged if unknown and all patients require a random glucose measurement.

More recently there has been considerable interest in the use of troponin (either T or I)

measurement in the diagnosis and management of the acute coronary syndromes. The troponins are proteins that regulate the interaction between actin and myosin in cardiac myocytes, and are highly sensitive and specific markers for myocardial cell injury. Troponin T has been found to be elevated in 30–50% of all patients with unstable angina.[49] In a prospective analysis of data from the GUSTO IIa trial, elevated troponin T levels were predictive of 30 day mortality.[50] A retrospective analysis of blood samples from the TIMI IIIb trial showed a similar relationship with troponin I.[51]

Coronary angiography
Anatomy

There is considerable heterogeneity among individuals presenting with unstable angina but if one considers the whole population of patients with this syndrome, the extent and severity of coronary disease is similar to that found in stable angina. There is, however, a correlation between the anatomical findings at angiography and the clinical presentation. Patients with long antecedent history of angina prior to the unstable episode, or of previous MI are more likely to have multivessel disease, whereas in those patients whose first manifestation of coronary artery disease is unstable angina, single vessel (usually involving the left anterior descending artery) disease is frequently found.[52]

If one considers all those patients with unstable angina who undergo angiography, up to 14% have no significant obstructive coronary disease, two-thirds have multivessel disease and approximately 10% have left main stem disease.[53] In the TIMI IIIa trial almost a third of those without significant coronary disease demonstrated abnormal filling patterns with the angiographic contrast media. Microvascular spasm with or without dysfunction has also been proposed as a possible mechanism.[54] The coronary lesion responsible for the episode of instability as in other acute coronary syndromes is frequently mild to moderately stenotic, with no correlation between the degree of stenosis and severity of clinical presentation, suggesting that plaque morphology and thrombus is important.

Plaque morphology

Complex lesion morphology (stenosis with irregular borders, overhanging edges and intracoronary thrombus) is found much more commonly in patients with unstable angina than in those with stable coronary disease. There is a correlation between the severity of clinical presentation and lesion morphology. Recurrent rest pain and refractory or post-infarction unstable angina are strongly associated with complex lesions and particularly intracoronary thrombus with reduced flow.[55]

Indications for angiography in patients with unstable angina

There is considerable geographic variation in the proportion of patients with acute coronary syndromes undergoing coronary angiography. One could argue that since the group as a whole has a significant incidence of either adverse cardiac events or recurrent ischaemia (especially early on), then all patients with a diagnosis of unstable angina should have coronary angiograms. As, in reality, such an approach would be impracticable and probably undesirable, it is necessary to identify those who are likely to benefit symptomatically or prognostically from revascularization or in whom diagnostic angiography is needed to clarify the diagnosis.

Natural history and prognosis

As we have already seen, Q-wave, non-Q-wave MI and unstable share a common pathogenesis. Up to 15% of patients with unstable angina may progress to MI and, of those patients admitted with acute MI, 30–60% experience unstable symptoms prior to presentation. Overall the risk of death from unstable angina is intermediate between that of stable angina and MI. The mortality from a single episode has been variously reported from between 4 and 14%. This probably reflects both in the broad range of patients with unstable angina and improvements in the management of this condition.

Mortality from an episode of unstable angina has been reported anywhere between 4 and 18% with lower mortality being quoted from more recent studies, possibly reflecting the improvements in the modern management of this condition.[56,57]

Recurrent episodes of ischaemia are also common—a prospective study of patients admitted to a single coronary care unit with unstable angina revealed that 35% of patients required revascularization, and the composite risk of death or readmission following a bout of unstable angina was 32%.[57] Furthermore, of those patients on an elective waiting list for angioplasty whose unstable angina had apparently settled, over half were either readmitted with MI or unstable angina, or the target vessels for angioplasty were found to have occluded.[58] Also angiographic follow-up of this population shows more progression of culprit lesions compared to patients with stable angina.

The early course in unstable angina is complicated and the risk of death and MI is highest in the first few months. There is evidence, however, to suggest that after the first year the risk of adverse events is similar to that in a population with stable coronary disease.

Risk stratification

As we have seen, patients with unstable angina have a variable prognosis and it is important to identify individuals at high risk of MI and other adverse outcomes. With resources being scarce, it is also helpful to identify those patients at low risk of subsequent events and to help them avoid prolonged hospitalization and perhaps unnecessary and expensive investigation.

Simple clinical and ECG variables are helpful in identifying high- and low-risk individuals. Clinical features indicative of high risk include post-infarction unstable angina, recurrent pain in hospital, the need for intravenous therapy and evidence of left ventricular dysfunction. ECG variables associated with high risk include transient ST depression with cardiac pain, and symmetrical anterior T wave inversion indicating proximal left anterior descending artery disease.

Low-risk individuals have no recurrent symptoms and a normal ECG. A negative maximal treadmill test points to a low risk of future events. Recent studies have suggested that troponin measurement gives further prognostic information.

Of those patients who come to angiography, left main stem disease, multivessel disease, depressed left ventricular function and complex culprit lesion morphology are all negative prognostic indicators.

References

1. Braunwald E, Mark DB, Jones RH et al, *Unstable Angina: Diagnosis and Management. Clinical Practice Guideline Number 1.* AHCPR Publication No. 94–0602. Agency for Health Care Policy and Research and the National Heart, Lung, and Blood Institute, Public Health Service, US Department of Health and Human Services; Rockville, MD, 1994.

2. Lewis HD Jr, Davis JW, Archibald DG et al, Protective effects of aspirin against acute myocardial infarction and death in men with unstable angina. Results of a Veterans Cooperative Study, *N Engl J Med* 1983; **309:** 396–403.

3. The RISC Group, Risk of myocardial infarction and death during treatment with low-dose aspirin and intravenous heparin in men with unstable coronary artery disease, *Lancet* 1990; **336:** 827–30.

4. The HINT Research Group, Early treatment of unstable angina in the coronary care unit. A randomized, double-blind, placebo-controlled comparison of recurrent ischaemia in patients treated with nifedipine or metoprolol or both, *Br Heart J* 1986; **56:** 400–13.

5. Chesebro JH, Badimon JJ, Platelet glycoprotein IIb/IIIa receptor blockade in unstable coronary disease, *N Engl J Med* 1998; **338:** 1539–41.

6. The PURSUIT Trial Investigators, Inhibition of platelet glycoprotein IIb/IIIa with eptifibatide in patients with acute coronary syndromes, *N Engl J Med* 1998; **339:** 436–43.

7. Braunwald E, Jones RH, Mark DB et al, Diagnosing and managing unstable angina, *Circulation* 1994; **90:** 613–22.

8. Crea F, Kaski JC, Maseri A, Key references on coronary artery spasm, *Circulation* 1994; **89:** 2442–6.

9. Braunwald E, Unstable angina. A classification, *Circulation* 1989; **80:** 410–14.

10. Calvin JE, Klein LW, VandenBerg BJ et al, Risk stratification in unstable angina. Prospective validation of the Braunwald classification, *JAMA* 1995; **273:** 136–41.

11. Van Miltenburg-van Zijl AJ, Simoons ML, Veerhoek RJ, Bossuyt PM, Incidence and follow-up of Braunwald subgroups in unstable angina pectoris, *J Am Coll Cardiol* 1995; **25:** 1286–92.

12. Bugiardini R, Borghi A, Pozzati A et al, Relation of severity of symptoms to transient myocardial ischemia and prognosis in unstable angina, *J Am Coll Cardiol* 1995; **25:** 597–604.

13. Chierchia S, Brunelli C, Simonetti I et al, Sequence of events in angina at rest. Primary reduction in coronary flow, *Circulation* 1980; **61:** 759–68.

14. Patel DJ, Knight CJ, Holdright DR et al, Pathophysiology of transient myocardial ischemia in acute coronary syndromes. Characterization by continuous ST segment monitoring, *Circulation* 1997; **95:** 1185–92.

15. Davies MJ, Thomas AC, Plaque fissuring – The cause of acute myocardial infarction, sudden ischaemic death and crescendo angina, *Br Heart J* 1985; **53:** 363–73.

16. Maseri A, L'Abbate A, Baroldi G, Coronary vasospasm as a possible cause of myocardial infarction. A conclusion based on the study of 'preinfarction' angina, *N Engl J Med* 1978; **299:** 1271–7.

17. Moise A, Theroux P, Taeymans Y, Unstable angina and progression of coronary atherosclerosis, *N Engl J Med* 1983; **309:** 685–9.

18. Falk E, Shah PK, Furster V, Coronary plaque disruption, *Circulation* 1995; **92**: 657–71.

19. Furster V, Badimon L, Badimon JJ, Chesebro JH, The pathogenesis of coronary artery disease and the acute coronary syndromes, *N Engl J Med* 1992; **326**: 242–50.

20. Zalewski A, Shi Y, Nardone D et al, Evidence for reduced fibrinolytic activity in unstable angina at rest. Clinical, biochemical, and angiographic correlates, *Circulation* 1991; **83**: 1685–91.

21. Mizuno K, Satomura K, Miyamoto A et al, Angioscopic evaluation of coronary artery thrombi in acute coronary syndromes, *N Engl J Med* 1992; **326**: 287–91.

22. Davies MJ, Thomas AC, Knapman PA, Hangartner JR, Intramyocardial platelet aggregation in patients with unstable angina suffering sudden ischemic cardiac death, *Circulation* 1986; **73**: 418–27.

23. Grande P, Grauholt AM, Madsen JK, Unstable angina pectoris. Platelet behavior and prognosis in progressive angina and intermediate coronary syndrome, *Circulation* 1990; **81**(Suppl I): I16–I19, discussion I22–I23.

24. Merlini PA, Bauer KA, Oltrona L et al, Persistent activation of coagulation mechanism in unstable angina and myocardial infarction, *Circulation* 1994; **90**: 61–8.

25. Kruskal JB, Commerford PJ, Franks JJ, Kirsch RE, Fibrin and fibrinogen-related antigens in patients with stable and unstable coronary artery disease, *N Engl J Med* 1987; **317**: 1361–5.

26. Schomig A, Neuman F-J, Kastrati A et al, A randomized comparison of antiplatelet and anticoagulant therapy after the placement of coronary artery stents, *N Engl J Med* 1996; **334**: 1084–91.

27. Willerson JT, Golino P, Eidt J et al, Specific platelet mediators and unstable coronary artery lesions. Experimental evidence and potential clinical implications, *Circulation* 1989; **80**: 198–205.

28. Qiu S, Theroux P, Marcil M, Solymoss BC, Plasma endothelin-1 levels in stable and unstable angina, *Cardiology* 1993; **82**: 12–19.

29. Maseri A, Sanna T, The role of plaque fissures in unstable angina: fact or fiction? *Eur Heart J* 1998; **19**(Suppl K): K2–K4.

30. Libby P, Molecular basis of the acute coronary syndromes, *Circulation* 1995; **91**: 2844–50.

31. Morrow DA, C-reactive protein and mortality in unstable angina, *J Am Coll Cardiol* 1998; **31**: 1460–5.

32. Liuzzo G, Biasucci LM, Gallimore R et al, Prognostic value of the acute phase proteins CRP and SAA in unstable angina and acute myocardial infarction, *N Engl J Med* 1994; **331**: 417–25.

33. Patel P, Mendall MA, Carrington D, Association of *Helicobacter pylori* and *Chlamydia pneumoniae* infections with coronary heart disease and cardiovascular risk factors, *BMJ* 1995; **311**: 711–14.

34. Danesh J, Wong Y, Ward M, Muir J, Chronic infection with *Helicobacter pylori*, *Chlamydia pneumoniae*, or cytomegalovirus. Population-based survey of coronary heart disease, *Heart* 1999; **81**: 245–7.

35. Gupta S, Leatham EW, Carrington D et al, Elevated *Chlamydia pneumoniae* antibodies, cardiovascular events, and azithromycin in male survivors of myocardial infarction, *Circulation* 1997; **96**: 404–7.

36. Theroux P, Furster V, Acute coronary syndromes, unstable angina, and non-Q wave

myocardial infarction, *Circulation* 1998; **97**: 1195–206.

37. Cannon CP, McCabe CH, Stone PH, The electrocardiogram predicts one year outcome of patients with unstable angina and non-Q wave myocardial infarction. Results from the TIMI III registry ancillary study, *J Am Coll Cardiol* 1997; **30**: 133–40.

38. Bosch X, Theroux P, Pelletier GB et al, Clinical and angiographic features and prognostic significance of early postinfarction angina with and without electrocardiographic signs of transient ischemia, *Am J Med* 1991; **91**: 493–501.

39. Murphy JJ, Connell PA, Hampton JR et al, Predictors of risk in patients with unstable angina admitted to a district general hospital, *Br Heart J* 1992; **67**: 395–401.

40. Holmvang L, Clemmensen P, Wagner G, Grande P, Admission standard electrocardiogram for early risk stratification in patients with unstable coronary artery disease not eligible for acute revascularization therapy. A TRIM substudy, *Am Heart J* 1999; **137**: 24–33.

41. Plotnick GD, Greene HL, Carliner NH et al, Clinical indicators of left main coronary artery disease in unstable angina, *Ann Intern Med* 1979; **91**: 149–53.

42. Haines DE, Raabe DS, Gundel WD, Wackers FJ, Anatomic and prognostic significance of new T wave inversion in unstable angina, *Am J Cardiol* 1983; **52**: 14–18.

43. De Zwaan C, Bär FW, Janssen JH, Angiographic and clinical characteristics of patients with unstable angina showing an ECG pattern indicating critical narrowing of the proximal LAD coronary artery. *Am Heart J* 1989; **117**: 657–65.

44. Nademanee K, Intarachot V, Josephson MA et al, Prognostic significance of silent myocardial ischemia in patients with unstable angina. *J Am Coll Cardiol* 1987; **10**: 1–9

45. Patel DJ, Holdright DR, Knight CJ et al, Early continuous ST monitoring in unstable angina. Prognostic value additional to the clinical characteristics and admission electrocardiogram, *Heart* 1996; **75**: 222–8.

46. Swahn E, Areskog M, Berglund U et al, Predictive importance of clinical findings and a predischarge exercise test in patients with suspected unstable coronary artery disease, *Am J Cardiol* 1987; **59**: 208–14.

47. Brown KA, Prognostic value of thallium-201 myocardial perfusion imaging in patients with unstable angina who respond to medical treatment, *J Am Coll Cardiol* 1991; **17**: 1053–7, erratum **18**: 889.

48. Stein JH, Neumann A, Preston LM et al, Improved risk stratification in unstable angina. Identification of patients at low risk for in-hospital cardiac events by admission echocardiography, *Clin Cardiol* 1998; **21**: 725–30.

49. Lindahl B, Venge P, Wallentin L, Relation between troponin T and the risk of subsequent cardiac events in unstable coronary artery disease. The FRISC study group, *Circulation* 1996; **93**: 1651–7.

50. Ohman EM, Armstrong PW, Christenson RH et al, Cardiac troponin T levels for risk stratification in acute myocardial ischemia. The GUSTO IIa Investigators, *N Eng J Med* 1996; **335**: 1333–41.

51. Antman EM, Tanasijevic MJ, Thompson B, Cardiac-specific troponin I levels to predict the risk of mortality in patients with acute coronary syndromes, *N Engl J Med* 1996; **335**: 1342–9.

52.   Hussain KM, Gould L, Barathan T et al,
      Arteriographic morphology and intracoronary
      thrombus in patients with unstable angina,
      non-Q wave myocardial infarction and stable
      angina pectoris, *Angiology* 1995; **46**: 181–9.

53.   Victor MF, Likoff MJ, Mintz GS, Likoff W,
      Unstable angina pectoris of new onset: a
      prospective clinical and arteriographic study
      of 75 patients, *Am J Cardiol* 1981; **47**:
      228–32.

54.   Diver DJ, Bier JD, Ferreira PE et al, Clinical
      and arteriographic characterization of patients
      with unstable angina without critical coronary
      arterial narrowing (from the TIMI-IIIA trial),
      Am J Cardiol 1994; **74**: 531–7.

55.   Dangas G, Mehran R, Wallenstein S et al,
      Correlation of angiographic morphology and

clinical presentation in unstable angina, *J Am
Coll Cardiol* 1997; **29**: 519–25.

56.   Gazes PC, Mobley EM Jr, Faris HM Jr et al,
      Preinfarction (unstable) angina. A prospective
      study – ten-year follow-up, *Circulation* 1973;
      48: 331–7.

57.   Cairns JA, Singer J, Gent M et al, One-year
      mortality outcomes of all coronary intensive
      care unit patients with acute myocardial
      infarction, unstable angina or other chest pain
      in Hamilton, Ontario, a city of 375,000
      people, *Can J Cardiol* 1989; **5**: 239–46.

58.   Chester M, Chen L, Kaski JC, Identification
      of patients at high risk for adverse coronary
      events while awaiting routine coronary
      angioplasty, *Br Heart J* 1995; **73**: 216–22.

Medical treatment of unstable angina

Kim Priestley

2

Introduction

Patients with unstable angina are at the watershed between angina pectoris and myocardial infarction. The aim of medical treatment is to control symptoms of myocardial ischaemia, and prevent progression to myocardial infarction and death. Anti-anginal therapy aims to optimize the balance between myocardial oxygen supply and demand, while antiplatelet and anticoagulant therapy limits thrombus formation. Anti-anginal agents have been used for many years in the symptomatic relief of ischaemic pain in unstable angina. Although they form conventional treatment in everyday clinical practice, few have been rigorously subjected to large, randomized, placebo-controlled trials. In contrast, the last 15 years has seen major developments in the use of antithrombotic agents in unstable angina. Well-designed and well-conducted clinical trials are available on which to base our clinical practice in this area. Once the diagnosis of unstable angina is suspected, treatment should be initiated as soon as possible. Patients should be admitted to hospital for bedrest and monitoring and managed whenever possible on a coronary care unit. All patients should have intravenous access secured, and receive adequate pain relief and supplemental oxygen therapy. Most patients with unstable angina will stabilize with optimal medical therapy. A small number of patients with refractory angina considered to be at high risk will require early coronary angiography and appropriate revascularization. This is discussed fully in subsequent chapters. The 30-day combined rate of death and non-fatal myocardial infarction for patients with unstable angina remains nearly 10%, despite therapy with aspirin, heparin or hirudin, beta-blockers, nitrates, calcium-channel blockers and revascularization.[1] Thus there is still room for improvement in the management of patients with unstable angina.

Anti-anginal therapy

Beta-blockers

Beta-blockers reduce oxygen demand by decreasing heart rate and myocardial contractility. They relieve symptoms of unstable angina and there is limited evidence that they may help prevent progression to myocardial infarction. In 1980 the Dutch HINT group[2] initiated a randomized, double-blind, placebo-controlled trial to assess the role of nifedipine and metoprolol (100 mg twice daily) in unstable angina. The main outcome event was recurrent ischaemia or myocardial infarction within 48 h. The results

suggested that in patients not already on a beta-blocker, metoprolol has a beneficial short-term effect. A later overview of four randomized, placebo-controlled trials of beta-blockers (propranolol, atenolol or metoprolol) in patients with 'threatened myocardial infarction' found that initial treatment with intravenous beta-blockers followed by oral treatment for a week reduced the risk of developing a myocardial infarct by about one-sixth.[3] Intravenous beta-blockers are seldom used in clinical practice, and initiation of beta-blockade with oral therapy has not been evaluated in large, prospective, randomized trials.

All patients presenting with unstable angina should receive a beta-blocker unless contraindicated. A number of different beta-blockers (propranolol, atenolol, metoprolol) have been used in small studies of patients with unstable angina and they all appear to exert similar effects. The evidence available from clinical trials favours an initial intravenous bolus to achieve rapid beta-blockade.

Calcium-channel blockers

Calcium-channel blockers are a heterogeneous group of drugs, most of which act on the L-type calcium channels in the heart or peripheral vasculature. Depending upon which calcium-channel blocker is chosen, they may reduce myocardial contractility, depress the formation and propagation of electrical impulses in the heart, and diminish coronary or systemic vascular tone. The dihydropyridines form the largest class of calcium-channel blockers and are typified by the drug nifedipine. Nifedipine acts principally on peripheral vascular smooth muscle, effecting a drop in peripheral vascular resistance and blood pressure with little direct myocardial effect. The Dutch HINT study[2] showed that patients receiving nifedipine alone had higher event rates than patients on placebo. However, when nifedipine was given to patients already on a beta-blocker, event rates were lower than in the placebo group. The higher incidence of myocardial infarction with nifedipine monotherapy was probably because of reflex tachycardia due to a decrease in blood pressure. Most non-dihydropyridine calcium-channel blockers, such as diltiazem and verapamil, have equal selectivity for myocardial and peripheral vascular channels, thus producing myocardial contractile depression and dilatation of resistance vessels. They also act on calcium channels in the sinus and atrioventricular nodes, producing a negative chronotropic effect and eliminating the harmful reflex tachycardia. A randomized, double-blind trial published in 1995 compared intravenous diltiazem with intravenous glyceryl trinitrate in 129 patients with unstable angina.[4] The doses of both drugs were titrated as necessary to the maximum allowed in the study. Over 48 h, diltiazem reduced the number of patients

with refractory angina and myocardial infarction to 12 (20%) versus 25 (41%), relative risk 0.49.

Short-acting dihydropyridine calcium-channel blockers such as nifedipine should be avoided in unstable angina. Diltiazem and verapamil should be reserved for patients with unstable angina in whom a beta-blocker is poorly tolerated or contraindicated. Both agents are, however, contraindicated in patients with significant left ventricular impairment or major disturbances of cardiac conduction. Verapamil should not be used concomitantly with a beta-blocker.

Nitrates

Although nitrates were among the first drugs used to treat patients with chest pain, their mechanisms of action remain poorly understood and there are few trials in unstable angina. Nitrates produce systemic venodilatation, which lowers preload, and vasodilatation of larger arteries, decreasing afterload. Both effects are additive in reducing myocardial oxygen demand. Myocardial perfusion is improved by dilatation of epicardial coronary vessels. A number of small studies have demonstrated the effectiveness of nitrates for both pain relief and prophylaxis of ischaemic episodes.[5,6] Sublingual nitroglycerin produces rapid relief of angina but remains effective for only 10–20 min. Oral nitrate preparations are effective for angina prophylaxis, having a more prolonged duration of effect, but their slow onset of action makes them less suitable for the treatment of patients with unstable symptoms. Continuous infusion of one of the intravenous nitrate preparations (isosorbide dinitrate 2–10 mg/h, or glyceryl trinitrate 10–200 µg/min) has several advantages in patients with unstable symptoms. They can be started at low dose and increased as necessary. The dose should be titrated against symptoms and the systolic blood pressure. Any unwanted side-effects of the drug resolve rapidly on stopping the infusion. Up to 25% of patients receiving intravenous nitrates complain of headache, which usually responds to simple analgesics such as paracetamol. Nitrate tolerance, with reduced clinical effect, has been reported with intravenous nitrates but is seldom a recognized problem in clinical practice. The intravenous preparation is continued until the patient's condition has stabilized, when an oral long-acting nitrate can be introduced, or until a definitive revascularization procedure is performed.

Antiplatelet therapy

Aspirin

Aspirin inhibits platelet cyclooxygenase-1 and the production of thromboxane A_2, thus preventing the second phase of platelet aggregation. A number of randomized, controlled trials have demonstrated that aspirin reduces both non-fatal myocardial infarction and cardiac deaths in patients with unstable angina, and is well tolerated. In 1983, the Veterans Administration Cooperative Study[7] reported on 1266 men with unstable angina, randomized within 48 h of admission to receive either 324 mg aspirin daily or placebo. The principal end-points were death and acute myocardial infarction. Aspirin reduced the combined incidence of death or myocardial infarction to 5.0%, as compared with 10.1% in the placebo group. Fatal or non-fatal myocardial infarction was 55% lower in the aspirin group; the reduction in mortality was of a similar magnitude (51%), but did not achieve statistical significance because of the relatively small numbers. At 1 year, the mean mortality rate in the aspirin group was 43% less than in the placebo group, although study drugs were discontinued at 12 weeks. Cairns et al[8] reported a study of 555 patients with unstable angina randomized within 8 days of admission to receive either aspirin (325 mg four times daily), sulfinpyrazone (200 mg four times daily), both or neither. Treatment and follow-up was for a mean of 18 months. This study recruited both male and female patients, like most subsequent studies. Aspirin reduced the primary end-point of cardiac death or non-fatal myocardial infarction by 30% on intention-to-treat analysis. Cardiac death alone was reduced by 56% with aspirin. No significant effect was observed with sulfinpyrazone. A later study by Theroux et al[9] randomized 479 patients on admission with unstable angina to receive either aspirin, heparin, both or neither. Aspirin was administered as 650 mg, immediately followed by 325 mg, twice daily. This was an acute-phase trial which ended when definitive treatment was selected after a mean of 6 days. Aspirin reduced the combined rate of fatal and non-fatal myocardial infarction by 72% as compared with placebo. Aspirin and heparin reduced the incidence of refractory angina, but not aspirin alone. Too few deaths occurred to allow meaningful analysis. In all three studies, side-effects of aspirin were relatively infrequent and minor, and withdrawal rates were similar in the aspirin and placebo groups.

It is recognized that the antiplatelet effects of aspirin are present even at low doses. The RISC Group[10] examined the benefits of low-dose aspirin and intravenous heparin in a randomized, double-blind, placebo-controlled study of 796 men with unstable angina or non-Q-wave myocardial infarction published in 1990. Aspirin 75 mg daily or placebo was administered within 72 h of admission and continued for at least 3 months. Patients were almost equally divided into those with unstable angina and those with non-Q-wave myocardial infarction. A similar response to aspirin treatment was observed in all subgroups. The event rates reported were for myocardial infarction or death at 5, 30 and 90 days. Low-dose aspirin reduced the event rate by 57–69% from day 5 onwards. Benefit in the first 5 days was only significant in the group receiving both aspirin and heparin. This may be explained by a time delay for low-dose aspirin (75 mg daily) to achieve platelet inhibition, as higher doses of aspirin have been shown to be effective acutely.[9] The randomized treatment was planned to continue for more than 12 months but the study was terminated prematurely on ethical grounds. The longer-term results were reported separately.[11] After 6 and 12 months of aspirin treatment, the risk of myocardial infarction or death was reduced by 54% and 48% respectively, thus retaining the gain obtained in the first 3 months. The major benefits of treatment were observed during the first 3 months of the study. Low-dose aspirin appeared to be as effective as higher doses in long-term use.[7,8]

Aspirin should be given to all patients without contraindications to aspirin therapy, as soon as possible after a diagnosis of unstable angina is made. The initial dose of aspirin should be high (e.g. 300 mg) and should be administered in a soluble or chewable form to achieve rapid platelet inhibition. Thereafter, low-dose aspirin (75 mg daily) appears to be as effective as treatment in higher doses and may be better tolerated. Aspirin should be continued indefinitely.

Ticlopidine and clopidogrel

The thienopyridines ticlopidine and clopidogrel are antiplatelet agents which do not block cyclooxygenase but interfere with ADP-mediated platelet activation and antagonize the interaction of fibrinogen with its platelet receptor, the membrane glycoprotein IIb/IIIa. Balsano et al,[12] 10 years ago, conducted a small open-label study of 652 patients with unstable angina randomized to either conventional therapy alone or conventional therapy combined with ticlopidine (250 mg twice daily for 6 months). Conventional therapy at the time did not include aspirin. The primary end-points were fatal or non-fatal myocardial infarction and vascular death. Ticlopidine reduced cardiac death by 46.8% and non-fatal myocardial infarction by 46.1%. The benefits of ticlopidine did not become apparent until after 15 days of therapy, consistent with the delayed effects of ticlopidine on platelet aggregation. The administration of ticlopidine was associated with minor adverse reactions, gastrointestinal disorders (5.1%) and skin reactions (1.9%). Neutropenia, the most serious side-effect reported with ticlopidine, did not occur in this particular study.

Ticlopidine is not at present licensed for use in the UK. It may, however, be an alternative to aspirin for secondary prevention in patients intolerant of aspirin. Clinical trials have reported a very similar reduction in cardiac death and non-fatal myocardial infarction to that obtained with aspirin. Whether ticlopidine has any value in the acute phase of unstable angina remains to be proven. Clopidogrel has a longer half-life than ticlopidine, allowing once-daily dosing, and also appears to be safer. Clopidogrel has not yet, however, been evaluated for the treatment of unstable angina.

Glycoprotein IIb/IIIa receptor antagonists

Aspirin is the gold standard antiplatelet agent, being simple to use, safe and cost-effective. It is, however, only a weak platelet inhibitor, affecting only one of the pathways to platelet aggregation, the cyclooxygenase pathway, leaving the other pathway intact. Alternative agents, the glycoprotein IIb/IIIa receptor antagonists, have been developed which block the final common pathway of platelet aggregation. Most data are from studies of angioplasty, but early work using these agents in unstable angina has been encouraging. In the CAPTURE study,[13] patients with refractory angina received standard therapy with aspirin plus heparin and were randomly assigned to either the glycoprotein IIb/IIIa inhibitor abciximab or placebo, starting 18–24 h before angioplasty and continued for 1 h after the procedure. The frequency of myocardial infarction before angioplasty was significantly lower in patients receiving abciximab than in those receiving placebo, 0.6% versus 2.1%. The so-called 4P studies (PRISM, PRISM-PLUS, PARAGON-A and PURSUIT) investigated the use of glycoprotein IIb/IIIa inhibitors in the medical management of unstable angina. Reviewed at a recent symposium, a meta-analysis of these trials, including a total of 17 997 patients, showed an 11% reduction in death or myocardial infarction.[14] In all these studies there was a small increase in bleeding complications in patients receiving the glycoprotein IIb/IIIa inhibitor, particularly if used in combination with heparin.

Abciximab (ReoPro) is the only glycoprotein IIb/IIIa inhibitor available outside clinical trials in the UK. It is licensed for use as an adjunct to heparin and aspirin for the prevention of ischaemic complications in high-risk patients undergoing percutaneous transluminal coronary angioplasty. Abciximab is a chimeric monoclonal antibody and should be used once only. Most other glycoprotien IIb/IIIa inhibitors under development are peptide or peptide-like mimetics and their relative lack of antigenicity offers advantages with respect to safety. The search is now on for an oral glycoprotein IIb/IIIa inhibitor

which is both effective and safe when administered long term. Until then, aspirin remains the antiplatelet agent of first choice.

Antithrombotic therapy
Unfractionated heparin

Heparin is a mixture of sulphated mucopolysaccharides which binds to antithrombin III. Activated antithrombin III inactivates factor Xa, thereby inhibiting coagulation. Heparin and activated antithrombin III inhibit thrombin-induced platelet aggregation. Heparin has been shown to reduce the incidence of myocardial infarction and both symptomatic and silent myocardial ischaemia in patients with unstable angina. In 1981, Telford and Wilson[15] reported a randomized, double-blind, placebo-controlled trial using heparin, atenolol or both in 214 patients admitted with unstable angina. Heparin was given by intravenous bolus injection every 6 h and continued for 7 days. Patients receiving heparin developed significantly fewer myocardial infarctions, and this benefit was maintained at 8-week follow-up. Theroux et al,[9] in their acute study, randomized 479 patients with unstable angina to aspirin, heparin, or both. Heparin was administered as an intravenous bolus of 5000 units followed by an infusion of 1000 units/h. The infusion was adjusted to maintain coagulation times

1.5–2 times control values. Heparin reduced the incidence of refractory angina by 63% as compared with placebo. The incidence of myocardial infarction was reduced in all three treatment groups but no statistical difference could be demonstrated between treatment groups. An additional 245 patients were then randomized to either aspirin or heparin to allow direct comparison in a larger study.[16] Myocardial infarction developed in 0.8% of patients in the heparin group and in 3.7% of patients in the aspirin group, thus showing a significant benefit of heparin over aspirin. Serneri et al[17] conducted a randomized, double-blind study of 97 patients with unstable angina refractory to conventional anti-anginal treatments. In the first part of the study, patients were randomized to receive either heparin infusion, heparin bolus or aspirin and then observed for up to 7 days. On the first day of treatment, heparin infusion significantly decreased the frequency of symptomatic angina (by 84–94%), episodes of silent ischaemia (by 71–77%) and the overall duration of ischaemia (by 81–86%). Heparin bolus and aspirin were not effective.

Heparin is thus beneficial during the acute phase in patients with unstable angina, and should be commenced as soon as possible. Evidence favours use of an intravenous bolus of 5000 units of heparin followed by an infusion of 1000 units/h adjusted to maintain a coagulation time 1.5–2 times control values.

In published trials, the duration of heparin therapy has varied from 2 to 7 days.

Additional studies have been performed to discover whether the combination of aspirin and heparin is superior to either agent alone. The ATACS trial[18] published in 1994 compared aspirin plus anticoagulation with aspirin alone in a randomized, open-label study of 214 patients admitted with unstable angina or non-Q-wave myocardial infarction. Aspirin was administered as a bolus of 162.5 mg followed by 162.5 mg daily. Heparin was administered as a loading bolus followed by an infusion to maintain the coagulation at twice control values for 3–4 days when patients were switched to warfarin. Treatment was continued for 12 weeks. Significant benefit was shown for combination therapy in the first 14 days. A primary event (recurrent angina, myocardial infarction or death) occurred in 10% of patients on combination therapy versus 27% of patients on aspirin alone. However, some of this early benefit was lost, and by the end of the study there was only a trend favouring combination therapy. A meta-analysis of six randomized trials comparing the use of aspirin and heparin with aspirin alone in patients with unstable angina was published in 1996.[19] All six trials demonstrated a trend towards improved outcome with the use of combination therapy versus aspirin alone. Overall, treatment with aspirin and heparin conferred a 33%

reduction in risk of myocardial infarction or death in patients with unstable angina versus aspirin alone. There was a small but non-significant increase in risk of bleeding in patients treated with both aspirin and heparin.

Current evidence favours the use of both aspirin and heparin at least for the first few days of treatment in patients with unstable angina. There are, however, a number of practical difficulties and limitations in the administration of unfractionated heparin. There is a wide variation in its anticoagulant effect, due to plasma protein binding and neutralization of anticoagulant activity by activated platelets. Even when closely monitored in a clinical study, more than 80% of the patients receiving heparin had coagulation times outside the target range.[20] There is a risk of heparin-induced thrombocytopenia, especially if treatment is prolonged beyond 5 days, and when unfractionated heparin is discontinued there often follows a rebound in clinical events.[21] This narrow risk–benefit profile of unfractionated heparin has led to a search for alternatives.

Low molecular weight heparins

Low molecular weight heparins (LMWHs) are produced from unfractionated heparin but are relatively selective inhibitors of factor Xa, via antithrombin III. Thrombin inhibition is less than that occurring with unfractionated heparin. LMWHs have several advantages over unfractionated heparin, which may lead to improved efficacy and safety. They are resistant to inhibition by platelet factor IV and have minimal protein binding, improving bioavailability and producing a more predictable anticoagulant response. As the effects of LMWHs are predictable, they can be given in a fixed, weight-adjusted dose without anticoagulant monitoring. Patients can administer the drug themselves using the subcutaneous route. There are a number of different LMWHs available, with differing ratios of inhibition of factor Xa to thrombin and thus potentially different biological profiles and efficacy. A single molecule of factor Xa stimulates the production of hundreds of thrombin molecules. Unfractionated heparin inhibits both factor Xa and thrombin in a ratio of 1 : 1, whereas for enoxaparin the ratio is 3 : 1. The early studies compared LMWHs and aspirin with aspirin alone. For example, the FRISC study[22] showed that dalteparin (120 IU/kg every 12 h subcutaneously) added to aspirin reduced the frequency of death and non-fatal myocardial infarction by 63% when compared with aspirin alone during the acute phase in patients with unstable angina or non-Q-wave myocardial infarction. Later studies compared LMWHs with unfractionated heparin. In the FRIC study[23] of unstable angina, all 1482 patients received aspirin but were then randomized in an open manner to receive either dalteparin or unfractionated heparin. The rate of death, myocardial infarction or recurrent angina during the first 6 days was equivalent in the two groups. This might reflect the dose of dalteparin used. The ESSENCE trial[24] was a randomized, double-blind study of 3171 patients with unstable angina (70%) or non-Q-wave myocardial infarction. Patients were randomized to receive either enoxaparin (1 mg/kg subcutaneously every 12 h plus aspirin or unfractionated heparin plus aspirin. Treatment was continued for between 2 and 8 days. The primary end-point of death, myocardial infarction or recurrent angina at 14 days occurred in 16.6% of patients receiving enoxaparin compared with 19.8% receiving unfractionated heparin. This difference was sustained at 30 days. It was also found that fewer enoxaparin-treated patients required revascularization procedures, and these benefits were obtained with no excess in major haemorrhagic complications. Follow-up of this cohort has now been extended to 1 year, and the benefits achieved at 14 days and 30 days were maintained. A study is now in progress looking at longer-term administration of enoxaparin to see if this confers further benefit. The TIMI 11B trial will compare enoxaparin for 43 days plus aspirin with unfractionated heparin for up to 8 days plus aspirin.

Enoxaparin plus aspirin thus appears to be clinically superior to unfractionated heparin plus aspirin in the acute phase of unstable angina. Enoxaparin is simpler to administer and does not require anticoagulant monitoring. Based on the ESSENCE data, we should be changing our practice to the use of enoxaparin in place of unfractionated heparin for the treatment of patients with unstable angina. Cost analysis of the UK subgroup from ESSENCE also shows that this would be a cost-effective measure.[25]

Hirudin

Thrombin has a major role in the pathogenesis of acute coronary thrombus. Heparin, the mainstay of antithrombin therapy, works indirectly, requiring antithrombin III as a cofactor, and is not effective against thrombin already bound to the fibrin clot. Hirudin, however, is a naturally occurring direct thrombin inhibitor which is currently being investigated in the treatment of acute coronary syndromes. Early angiographic studies circa 1994 in patients with unstable angina showed hirudin to be superior to heparin in achieving angiographic improvement of the culprit arterial lesion.[20] A later, much larger, study compared hirudin (0.1 mg/kg bolus followed by 0.1 mg/kg per hour infusion) with heparin in 12 142 patients with a variety of acute coronary syndromes.[1] The clinical outcomes at 30 days were only marginally better with hirudin, and this was offset by a higher incidence of moderate bleeding with hirudin. The OASIS pilot study[26] compared two doses of hirudin with heparin in the acute treatment of patients with unstable angina or suspected acute myocardial infarction. Study infusions were continued when possible for 72 h. The higher dose of hirudin (0.4 mg/kg bolus followed by 0.15 mg/kg per hour infusion) resulted in a significant reduction in ischaemic events at 7 days compared with heparin. Minor bleeding was significantly increased in patients receiving either dose of hirudin. After discontinuation of study treatments, there was a rebound in ischaemic events in all treatment groups which attenuated some of the early difference compared with heparin.

These preliminary studies suggest that hirudin is likely to be more effective than heparin in preventing ischaemic events in patients with unstable angina but the increase in bleeding complications is a concern. Definitive evidence from larger trials is awaited, and the main OASIS hirudin data will be available shortly.

Oral anticoagulants

Oral anticoagulants antagonize the effects of vitamin K and take at least 48–72 h for the anticoagulant effect to develop, making them unsuitable for use during the acute phase of unstable angina. It is, however, recognized that although short-term antithrombotic treatments are beneficial in reducing ischaemic events, there still appears to be a delayed excess of such events when these agents are discontinued, and patients may benefit from more prolonged treatment. Current studies are investigating different strategies for providing longer-term antithrombotic treatment. One such strategy is to follow short-term intravenous treatment with long-term warfarin. However, at present there is no evidence to support the use of oral anticoagulants in patients with unstable angina.

Thrombolytic therapy

Thrombolytic drugs activate plasminogen to form plasmin, which degrades fibrin and thus lyses thrombi. In addition to these clot-dissolving properties, thrombolytic therapy also has procoagulant actions. Fibrin-bound thrombin is exposed and this is a potent stimulus of rethrombosis. Thrombolytic therapy also activates platelets directly. This Yin and Yang of thrombolytic therapy was evident in the TIMI IIIB[27] randomized trial of alteplase versus placebo in 1473 patients with unstable angina or non-Q-wave myocardial infarction. All patients were treated with bedrest, anti-ischaemic medications, aspirin and heparin. At 6 weeks, an unfavourable outcome (death, non-fatal myocardial infarction or failure of initial therapy) occurred in 54.2% of the patients given alteplase and 55.5% of those given placebo. Those patients with unstable angina had a higher occurrence of death or myocardial infarction by 42 days if treated with alteplase than if treated with placebo, 9.1% versus 5.0% respectively. There was also a trend towards an increased incidence of intracranial haemorrhage in patients receiving thrombolysis.

Therefore, thrombolytic therapy has no place in the routine treatment of patients with unstable angina.

New treatments under study

Potassium-channel activators

The potassium-channel activators form a new class of drugs with both arterial and venous vasodilating properties. Nicorandil is the first drug in this group to be licensed for clinical use in the UK and is indicated for the prophylaxis and treatment of stable angina. There have been a few small studies using intravenous nicorandil in unstable angina, and early results appear encouraging. A recent pilot study randomized 245 patients with unstable angina on conventional treatment to the addition of oral nicorandil or placebo.[28] Patients receiving nicorandil had fewer episodes of transient myocardial ischaemia on

ST segment Holter monitoring. The results of larger randomized clinical trials are awaited.

Antibiotic therapy

Evidence is accumulating that microbial pathogens such as *Chlamydia pneumoniae* and *Helicobacter pylori* may play a significant role in coronary artery disease. The randomized trial of roxithromycin (an antichlamydial macrolide antibiotic) in non-Q-wave coronary syndromes (ROXIS) pilot study[29] included 202 patients with unstable angina or non-Q-wave myocardial infarction. All patients received conventional therapy and were then randomly allocated to either roxithromycin (150 mg twice daily) or placebo for 30 days. Roxithromycin was associated with a significant reduction in clinical end-point rates (ischaemic death, acute myocardial infarction, and severe recurrent ischaemia). Larger-scale studies are now required to confirm these preliminary observations.

Secondary prevention

Patients with unstable angina who have survived the acute phase to hospital discharge remain at higher risk of recurrent events for at least the first 3 months and probably beyond. Low-dose aspirin has been shown to have a protective effect for at least 3 months, and in the absence of side-effects should probably be continued indefinitely.[11] Several studies are now in progress examining ways of maintaining antithrombotic therapy over this time period. Longer-term use of the LMWHs is one option which is currently being investigated, since these drugs are simple to use and can be self-administered. Aggressive cholesterol-lowering therapy may also be important in secondary prevention. The LIPID study[30] was a double-blind, randomized, placebo-controlled study in over 9000 patients with ischaemic heart disease and total cholesterol levels between 4.0 and 7.0 mmol/L which compared pravastatin (40 mg/day) with placebo. Patients had a history of myocardial infarction or hospitalization for unstable angina (36%). The study was stopped early because of significant benefits in the pravastatin group. Results show a reduction in cardiac death, myocardial infarction and the need for coronary bypass surgery in patients receiving pravastatin. The effects of treatment were similar for all predefined subgroups. These results suggest that patients should receive appropriate cholesterol-lowering treatment.

Future directions

The management of patients with unstable angina is evolving rapidly. The armamentarium of anti-anginal therapies has recently increased with the addition of the potassium-channel activators. Antiplatelet therapy now includes glycoprotein IIb/IIIa inhibitors, and oral agents are currently being evaluated in clinical trials. Antithrombotic therapy has advanced following the introduction of the LMWHs and direct thrombin inhibitors. New therapeutic avenues such as antibiotic treatment are being explored. There are interesting times ahead for all those involved in the clinical management of patients with unstable angina.

References

1. The global use of strategies to open occluded coronary arteries (GUSTO) IIb Investigators, A comparison of recombinant hirudin with heparin for the treatment of acute coronary syndromes, *N Engl J Med* 1996; **335**: 775–82.

2. Report of the Holland Interuniversity Nifedipine/Metoprolol Trial (HINT) research group, Early treatment of unstable angina in the coronary care unit: a randomised, double blind, placebo controlled comparison of recurrent ischaemia in patients treated with nifedipine or metoprolol or both, *Br Heart J* 1986; **56**: 400–13.

3. Yusaf S, The use of beta blockers in the acute phase of myocardial infarction. In: Califf RM, Wagner GS, eds, *Acute Coronary Care* (Martinus Nijhoff Publishing: Boston 1986) 73–88.

4. Bobel EJAM, Hautvast RWM, van Gilst WH et al, Randomised, double-blind trial of intravenous diltiazem versus glyceryl trinitrate for unstable angina pectoris, *Lancet* 1995; **346**: 1653–7.

5. Mikolich JR, Nicoloff NB, Robinson PH, Logue RB, Relief of refractory angina with continuous intravenous infusion of nitroglycerin, *Chest* 1980; **77**: 375–9.

6. Curfman GD, Heinsimer JA, Lozner EC, Fung H-L, Intravenous nitroglycerin in the treatment of spontaneous angina pectoris: a prospective, randomized trial, *Circulation* 1983; **67**: 276–82.

7. Lewis HD Jr, Davis JW, Archibald DG et al, Protective effects of aspirin against acute myocardial infarction and death in men with unstable angina. Results of a Veterans Cooperative Study, *N Engl J Med* 1983; **309**: 396–403.

8. Cairns JA, Gent M, Singer J et al, Aspirin, sulfinpyrazone, or both in unstable angina. Results of a Canadian Multicenter Trial, *N Engl J Med* 1985; **313**: 1369–75.

9. Theroux P, Ouimet H, McCans J et al, Aspirin, heparin, or both to treat acute unstable angina, *N Engl J Med* 1988 **319**: 1105–11.

10. The RISC Group, Risk of myocardial infarction and death during treatment with low dose aspirin and intravenous heparin in men with unstable coronary artery disease, *Lancet* 1990; **336**: 827–30.

11. Wallentin LC and the research group on instability in coronary artery disease in Southeast Sweden, Aspirin (75 mg/day) after an episode of unstable coronary artery disease: long-term effects on the risk for myocardial infarction, occurrence of severe angina and the need for revascularization, *J Am Coll Cardiol* 1991; **18**: 1587–93.

12. Balsano F, Rizzon P, Violi F et al, Antiplatelet treatment with ticlopidine in unstable angina: a controlled multicenter clinical trial, *Circulation* 1990; **82**: 17–26.

13. The CAPTURE investigators, Randomised placebo-controlled trial of abciximab before and during coronary intervention in refractory unstable angina: the CAPTURE study, *Lancet* 1997; **349**: 1429–35.

14. White H, New approaches to the modern management of unstable angina, *Br J Cardiol* 1998; 5(suppl 3): 58–9.

15. Telford AM, Wilson C, Trial of heparin versus atenolol in prevention of myocardial infarction in intermediate coronary syndrome, *Lancet* 1981; **8232**: 1225–8.

16. Theroux P, Waters D, Qui S et al, Aspirin versus heparin to prevent myocardial infarction during the acute phase of unstable angina, *Circulation* 1993; **88**: 2045–8.

17. Serneri GGN, Gensini GF, Poggesi L et al, Effect of heparin, aspirin or alteplase in reduction of myocardial ischaemia in refractory unstable angina, *Lancet* 1990; **335**: 615–18.

18. Cohen M, Adams PC, Parry G et al, Combination antithrombotic therapy in unstable rest angina and non-Q-wave infarction in nonprior aspirin users: primary end points analysis from the ATACS trial, *Circulation* 1994; **89**: 81–8.

19. Oler A, Whooley MA, Oler J, Grady D, Adding heparin to aspirin reduces the incidence of myocardial infarction and death in patients with unstable angina: a meta-analysis, *JAMA* 1996; **276**: 811–12.

20. Topol EJ, Fuster V, Harrington RA et al, Recombinant hirudin for unstable angina pectoris: a multicenter, randomised angiographic trial, *Circulation* 1994; **89**: 1557–66.

21. Theroux P, Waters D, Lam J et al, Reactivation of unstable angina after the discontinuation of heparin, *N Eng J Med* 1992; **327**: 141–5.

22. The FRISC Study Group, Low molecular weight heparin during instability in coronary artery disease, *Lancet* 1996; **347**: 561–8.

23. Klein W, Buchwald A, Hillis SE et al, Comparison of low-molecular-weight heparin with unfractionated heparin acutely and with placebo for 6 weeks in the management of unstable coronary artery disease: fragmin in unstable coronary artery disease study, *Circulation* 1997; **96**: 61–8.

24. Cohen M, Demers C, Gurfinkel EP et al, A comparison of low-molecular-weight heparin with unfractionated heparin for unstable coronary artery disease, *N Eng J Med* 1997; **337**: 447–52.

25. Fox KAA, Bosanquet N, Assessing the UK cost implications of the use of low molecular weight heparin in unstable coronary artery disease, *Br J Cardiol* 1998; **5**: 92–105.

26. Organization to Assess Strategies for Ischemic Syndromes (OASIS) Investigators, Comparison of the effects of two doses of recombinant hirudin compared with heparin in patients with acute myocardial ischaemia without ST elevation: a pilot study, *Circulation* 1997; **96**: 769–77.

27. The TIMI IIIB Investigators, Effects of tissue plasminogen activator and a comparison of early invasive and conservative strategies in unstable angina and non-Q-wave myocardial infarction, *Circulation* 1994; **89**: 1545–56.

28. Patel DJ, Purcell HJ, Fox KM, Cardioprotection by opening of the K(ATP) channel in unstable angina. Is this a clinical manifestation of myocardial preconditioning? Results of a randomized study with nicorandil. CESAR 2 investigation. Clinical European studies in angina and revascularization, *Eur Heart J* 1999; **20**: 51–7.

29. Gurfinkel E, Bozovich G, Daroca A et al, for the ROXIS Study Group, Randomised trial of roxithromycin in non-Q-wave coronary syndromes: ROXIS pilot study, *Lancet* 1997; **350**: 404–7.

30. The Long-Term Intervention with Pravastatin in Ischaemic Distress (LIPID) Study Group, Prevention of cardiovascular events and death with pravastatin in patients with coronary heart disease and a broad range of initial cholesterol levels, *N Engl J Med* 1998; **339**: 1349–57.

Unstable angina: cardiac catheterization and findings

Rosemary A Rusk and Antoinette Kenny

3

Introduction

The aim of cardiac catheterization in patients with unstable angina is to obtain detailed anatomical information, thereby allowing assessment of prognosis and selection of a long-term management strategy. The procedure is usually helpful in choosing between medical therapy, percutaneous transluminal coronary angioplasty or coronary artery bypass surgery as the line of future management. Patients with contraindications to revascularization and patients who do not wish to consider interventional therapy should not undergo diagnostic catheterization.

Indications

There are different approaches regarding the indications and optimal timing of cardiac catheterization for unstable angina. The Agency for Health Care Policy and Research (AHCPR) Clinical Practice guidelines outline two different strategies, namely an early invasive strategy and an early conservative strategy.[1]

Early invasive strategy

All hospitalized patients with unstable angina and without contraindications receive cardiac catheterization within 48 h of presentation.

Early conservative strategy

Cardiac catheterization is performed on hospitalized patients with unstable angina if they have one or more of the following high-risk indicators. All other patients receive medical management and undergo cardiac catheterization only when medical management fails. The high-risk indicators include:

- persistent or recurrent pain/ischaemia
- functional study indicating high risk
- prior revascularization
- congestive cardiac failure or estimated ejection fraction less than 50%
- malignant ventricular arrhythmia.

These guidelines are based partly on the results of the TIMI-IIIB trial.[2] This trial randomized 1473 patients with unstable angina or non-Q-wave myocardial infarction admitted within 24 h of chest pain. The study had a 2 × 2 factorial design comparing tissue plasminogen activator versus placebo and an early invasive versus an early conservative strategy. The early invasive strategy (early coronary angiography followed by revascularization) was compared with the early conservative strategy (coronary angiography followed by revascularization if initial medical therapy failed) in terms of a composite end-point including death, myocardial infarction or an unsatisfactory symptom-limited exercise stress test at 6 weeks. In the early invasive arm, the revascularization rate at 6 weeks was 61%. Of the patients assigned to the conservative (non-catheterization) strategy, 60% required catheterization primarily for failure of initial therapy and the revascularization rate was 49%. There was no difference in the primary end-point between the two groups but the average length of initial hospitalization, along with the incidence and days of rehospitalization and level of medication, were lower in the early invasive strategy. Therefore, early coronary arteriography followed by revascularization, if coronary anatomy is suitable and there are no contraindications, may be the more appropriate approach for patients admitted to a centre with facilities for angioplasty and surgery on site. Further studies are ongoing, also aimed at investigating whether an early interventional approach improves outcome within a modern clinical setting.

Although, partly from a logistical and a practical point of view, the early invasive policy is not practised in all hospitals, the policy for proceeding promptly in patients with high-risk indicators is well established. In patients who respond initially to medical therapy or in whom the indications for intervention are less clear, non-invasive investigation is often used for further risk stratification. Patients with angina at a low exercise workload, marked ischaemic changes or exercise-induced hypotension on exercise stress testing, warrant coronary arteriography.[3] Patients who have not experienced rest pain, who have new-onset angina with an onset more than 2 weeks earlier or those with a normal or unchanged electrocardiogram during pain and who have settled on medical treatment, have been identified as being at a low risk for cardiac events on continued medical therapy. If these patients are asymptomatic on medical therapy and do not have a high-risk stress test, they may be followed without coronary arteriography with a low incidence of adverse cardiac events.[4]

The practice of selecting patients for angiography in different types of hospitals has been examined. Van Miltenburg-van Zijl and colleagues looked at the management strategy applied to patients with unstable angina both in a centre with and in one without in-house angiography. The clinical characteristics identified as important predictors for proceeding to angiography were similar in both centres. These included younger age group, male gender, progressive onset of angina, multiple episodes of pain, level of medication and abnormal ST-T segments at baseline or ECG changes during pain. However, in spite of this, angiography was performed more often in the presence of on-site angiography facilities (43% versus 25%) and the decision to proceed was made earlier. The more restricted use of angiography in the community hospital did not result in selecting a subset of patients with more advanced coronary disease, and the overall survival and infarct-free survival were the same in the two hospitals over a 6-month period.[5]

Pattern of disease

When patients with unstable angina, regardless of subgroup, are considered, coronary angiography shows a rather similar distribution of single-, double- and triple-vessel disease as in patients with chronic stable angina. Fig. 3.1 shows that three-vessel disease is found in approximately 40%, double-vessel disease in approximately 20%, left main stem stenosis in around 20% (higher than in patients with stable angina), single-vessel disease in around 10% and no significant obstruction in the remaining 10%.[4] Also, as in stable angina, the left anterior descending coronary artery is the most commonly affected vessel.

However, the diagnosis of unstable angina encompasses many subgroups, including angina at rest, post-myocardial infarction angina, accelerating or crescendo angina and

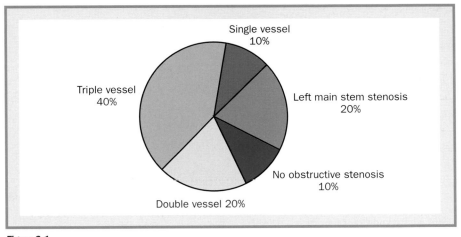

Figure 3.1
Distribution of number of vessels involved in patients presenting with unstable angina.

new-onset angina. Also, the pattern of disease seen at angiography changes when the duration of the history of angina is considered. Patients in whom unstable angina presents superimposed on a history of stable angina often have multivessel disease. In contrast, if unstable angina is the initial presentation of coronary artery disease, approximately 50% of cases have single-vessel disease and less than 20% three-vessel disease. Patients with new onset of rest pain may also only have disease of one coronary artery. These data have important implications in terms of assessing patients as potential revascularization candidates. Patients with crescendo angina on a background of stable angina tend to have left main stem disease or multivessel coronary obstruction and are most commonly treated with coronary artery bypass grafting. Patients with new-onset angina, who frequently have single-vessel disease, are often amenable to angioplasty.

In the group of patients with a diagnosis of unstable angina but normal coronary arteries on angiography or minimal disease, causes such as coronary spasm, spontaneous lysis of a coronary thrombus, abnormalities of the microvascular circulation or the presence of a lesion overlooked on arteriography may be responsible. Although Prinzmetal originally described a syndrome of focal coronary spasm that occurred at the site of a fixed atherosclerotic narrowing,[6] it is now accepted that spasm can occur at sites that are minimally diseased or angiographically completely normal. No severe obstructive lesion is found in approximately one-third of patients with variant angina, defined as angina occurring at rest and associated with transient ST elevation.[4] In some patients, however, the diagnosis of angina may be incorrect and there may be a non-coronary cause for their symptoms.

Distinguishing features between unstable and stable lesions

Although we know that traditional analysis of coronary arteriograms in terms of the number of vessels involved or the severity of disease is not particularly helpful in distinguishing unstable angina from the stable syndrome, it is now established that the two syndromes can be reliably differentiated in most cases by the angiographic morphology of the lesion. When the angiographic findings in patients with unstable angina and stable angina are compared, the frequency of complex lesions and the presence of intracoronary thrombus is higher in the former group.[7] These aspects are discussed in more detail.

Morphology of lesions

Background

The development of unstable angina may be associated with a change in coronary anatomy due to one or more of the following:

- plaque rupture
- coronary thrombosis
- coronary spasm.

Although stable and unstable angina do not differ in the number of diseased vessels, they can often be differentiated on the basis of angiographic morphology due to the role played by plaque rupture and coronary thrombosis. Lesion morphology was first described in unstable angina by Levin and Fallon, who carried out an autopsy study and visually inspected plane film post-mortem angiograms obtained in coronary vessels dissected free from the heart.[8] They found that lesions with irregular borders and intraluminal lucencies on angiography often demonstrated atherosclerotic plaque disruption or partially occlusive thrombi (79% of cases compared with only 11% of lesions with angiographically smooth borders).

Types of lesions

Similar irregularities of the arterial lumen to those documented in post-mortem angiograms can be seen on coronary angiograms obtained from patients with unstable angina. Morphology should be determined in orthogonal views in projections that avoid foreshortening of the lesion or overlap of the vessel.

The angiographic features of complex coronary lesions in unstable angina were initially described by Ambrose et al.[9] They described lesions as concentric stenoses which were symmetrical narrowings with smooth or only slightly irregular borders or eccentric stenoses. Eccentric lesions were asymmetrical and could be identified qualitatively by one or more of the following features:

- eccentricity
- narrow neck
- overhanging edges or irregular borders.

Their initial classification of lesions is depicted in Fig. 3.2. They classified unstable angina-producing lesions as type II eccentric lesions, identified by eccentric lesions with a narrow neck, overhanging edges or irregular borders. These are now referred to as complex stenoses.

In the American College of Cardiology/American Heart Association classification for coronary angioplasty, simple, concentric lesions are classified as type A.

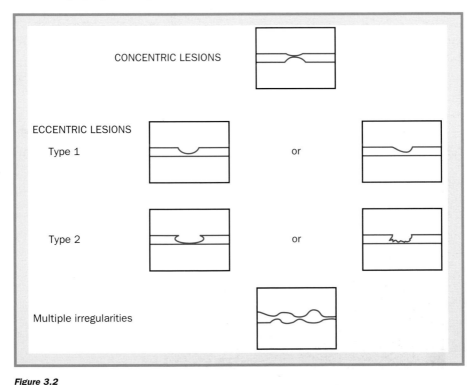

Figure 3.2
Angiographic classification of lesion morphology adapted from Ambrose et al.[13]

Complex lesions are further subdivided into moderately complex (type B) and complex (type C), differentiated primarily on the basis of length, degree of angulation and also the tortuosity of the proximal segment.[10]

In spite of coronary angioscopy and endovascular ultrasound studies stressing the limitations of angiography, it remains the only widely used diagnostic test in clinical practice.[11] Angiographic quantitative assessment of lesion eccentricity has been described[12] but the lesions are still most commonly interpreted visually. Although analysis of arterial borders by, for example, automated edge detection gives a more objective assessment of lesion irregularity, it does not incorporate an assessment of filling defects within the borders of the lesion.

Incidence of complex stenoses

Fig. 3.3 shows a complex stenosis in a patient presenting with unstable angina. It is now well established that patients with unstable angina have a high incidence of complex lesions. In the study by Ambrose et al, some or all of the features of complex stenoses were found in 54% of obstructive lesions in patients with unstable angina, compared with 7% in patients with stable angina.[9] In the same group, this type of lesion was found in 71% of

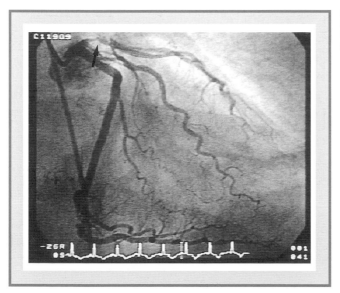

Figure 3.3
Complex stenosis proximally in the left anterior descending coronary artery.

angina-producing coronary arteries in those with unstable angina but in only 16% of arteries in those with stable angina. Concentric lesions were more frequent in patients with stable angina. These findings have been confirmed in subsequent studies.

Aetiological role of complex lesions in unstable angina

The appearance of a complex lesion is caused by an eccentric bulge into the lumen of the vessel and probably represents plaque disruption or a partially occlusive thrombus or both. A temporary decrease in coronary perfusion secondary to these plaques with or without superimposed platelet thrombi or altered vasomotor tone appears to be a major cause of unstable angina. Culprit lesions in unstable angina have been shown to exhibit greater vasoconstrictive potential in comparison with stable coronary artery lesions.[14]

Intracoronary thrombus can sometimes hide plaque disruption or fissuring, thereby disguising the appearance of the plaque and making it appear smooth. Evidence for this comes from studies of patients who have had thrombolytic therapy for acute myocardial infarction. Immediately following thrombolysis, coronary lesions often appear smooth, presumably because there is still a coating of thrombus on the inside of the vessel. Several days following infarction, however, the ulceration can be clearly seen.[15] Interestingly, Wilson et al also reported that lesions associated with recent infarction were significantly longer than those in stable angina. Although the lesions causing unstable angina were longer than those in stable cases, the difference was not significant. They proposed that residual intraluminal thrombus might have artifactually increased the apparent length of the lesion.[15]

Not all lesions associated with unstable angina are complex. In some cases, the development of unstable symptoms may occur due to transient increases in myocardial oxygen demand or other supply-related variables, such as coronary spasm or the development of anaemia rather than fissuring or disruption of a plaque with superimposed thrombosis. In these patients, the presence of a complex plaque may therefore not be required in the development of instability. It is estimated that alterations in perfusion and myocardial oxygen supply probably account for 67% of episodes of unstable angina, the remaining episodes probably being due to transient increases in demand for myocardial oxygen.[16]

Angiographic stenosis progression in patients with angina

Since the identification of complex lesions, the evolution of stenosis morphology in angina has been studied. Sequential studies in patients undergoing angiography before and after development of unstable angina have shown that the transition to the unstable state is associated with progression of coronary artery stenosis in about 75% of cases[7,17] and that the new unstable lesions have a specific morphology that has been described. Interestingly, in the study of Ambrose et al the majority of lesions (72%) with significant progression had shown insignificant disease at the time of first catheterization. In the unstable group, it was also noted that 71% of lesions that had progressed to a significant, non-occluded stenosis were complex in nature at repeat catheterization. In contrast, complex stenoses were not present in any vessels with disease progression in the stable group.[13]

Progression of disease is therefore very common in the acute presentation of unstable angina, with many of the lesions progressing from previously insignificant stenoses. A complex lesion is the most common configuration of coronary lesion in this type of progression. On the basis of histological studies, lesion progression in unstable angina is thought to result from remodelling and organization of plaque haemorrhage or from repeated subclinical cycles of rupture, haemorrhage and organization.[11]

Prognostic significance of lesion morphology

Angiographic morphology has been shown to be of relevance with regard to the risk of adverse coronary events. Available evidence suggests that complex stenoses may significantly alter the prognosis of the patient. Studies have looked at adverse coronary events both before and after discharge of patients hospitalized with an episode of unstable angina.

In-hospital events
In patients with unstable angina, angiographically complex stenoses have been shown to predict subsequent in-hospital instability.[18,19] In a study by Freeman et al, in-hospital cardiac events, including death, myocardial infarction and urgent revascularization, were more frequent in patients with complex coronary morphology. Fifty-five per cent of patients who suffered an adverse cardiac event had complex lesion morphology, compared with 31% in the uncomplicated group.[20] However, multiple regression analysis showed that complex coronary morphology was not independently predictive of cardiac events, and the best angiographic predictor was, in fact, the presence of intracoronary thrombus. Detection and relevance of coronary thrombus is discussed in the following section. It is of interest that, in Freeman's study, the

incidence of complex coronary morphology was not altered by whether angiography was performed immediately or later during admission for unstable angina.

Natural history of complex morphology post-discharge

Complex stenoses have also been associated with future disease progression. Kaski et al looked at features associated with rapid disease progression in patients awaiting elective coronary angioplasty. Patients had repeat arteriography at 8 ± 3 month follow-up — immediately preceding angioplasty or after an acute coronary event. Morphological appearance was found to be an independent factor in determining stenosis progression. Complex lesions progressed more than smooth stenoses, in patients presenting with stable or unstable angina (22% versus 4%, $p = 0.002$), and acute coronary events occurred in a significantly greater number of patients in whom stenoses had progressed.[21] Chen et al showed that in unstable patients who stabilized medically and were discharged from hospital, subsequent short-term stenosis progression and coronary events were common.[22] Disease progression during a mean interval of 8 months was demonstrated in 32% of patients who had been hospitalized with unstable angina, compared with 16% in patients with stable angina. During the follow-up period, 31% of this group had an acute coronary event (further episode of

unstable angina or acute myocardial infarction). Progression of the culprit stenosis was demonstrated in 54% of cases. Disease progression was significantly more common in complex lesions, and complex morphology and unstable angina were predictive factors for progression of culprit stenoses. It would therefore appear that complex stenosis morphology is a predictor of poor outcome in patients with unstable angina who have stabilized on medical therapy.

Intracoronary thrombus

Over the past few decades, the pathogenesis and pathophysiology of acute coronary syndromes have been extensively investigated. Pathological studies in patients who have succumbed to acute ischaemic syndromes have shown that the causative major plaque disruptions are complicated by thrombosis in most cases.[23] This has led to realization of the contributory role of intracoronary thrombosis in a large proportion of patients with unstable angina. The next section discusses angiographic detection of intracoronary thrombus and its implications.

Definition and detection

There still is no standardized angiographic definition of intracoronary thrombus. It is also generally accepted that distinguishing it from a complex lesion may be difficult. Definitions commonly used include:[24]

- the presence of a smooth central filling defect surrounded by contrast material seen in multiple projections, in the absence of calcification within the defect, and with or without persistent staining of the intraluminal material
- contrast medium staining at the site of an abrupt occlusion of a vessel.

The most specific angiographic hallmark of intracoronary thrombus is the presence of a globular filling defect, completely surrounded by contrast material and usually located distal to the point of the most severe stenosis.[25] When the lesion is eccentric and associated with contrast retention, there have been reports of thrombolytic intervention being unsuccessful, suggesting that these lesions may represent areas of microvascular channels rather than thrombus.[26]

Certain angiographic features, including stenosis severity, acuteness of the stenosis angle and the presence of a branch originating within the stenosis, are known to be associated with a higher risk of thrombosis.[27]

Fig. 3.4a shows intracoronary thrombus represented by a filling defect just distal to a severe stenosis in the right coronary artery (RCA). It was seen to embolize downstream during the course of the study (Fig. 3.4b).

Other methods to visualize coronary thrombi
The ability of visual assessment of coronary arteriograms to detect coronary thrombus remains unknown. It is known that its ability is limited compared with other imaging modalities, as it only provides a silhouette of lesion edges. Observations made using flexible fibreoptic angioscopes suggest that coronary mural thrombus is present in virtually all patients with unstable angina, even when it is not detected by angiography.[28] The thrombi seen in association with unstable angina typically have a greyish-white appearance which differs from the reddish thrombi seen with acute myocardial infarction. It is understandable that a thin-layered thrombus described in autopsy specimens may not be seen angiographically if it is adjacent to atherosclerotic lesions.[29] Interestingly, it has been found that intravascular ultrasound has difficulty in distinguishing thrombus from echolucent soft plaque.[30,31]

Even though intracoronary thrombus may be missed on angiography, it has been shown that when it is detected in patients with unstable angina, it has important prognostic and therapeutic implications.

Incidence

In unstable angina
The documented incidence of intracoronary thrombi at angiography in unstable angina

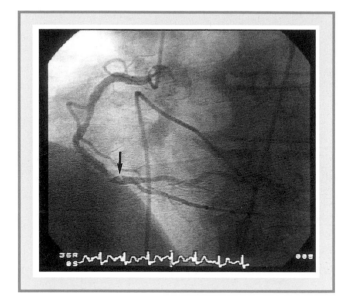

Figure 3.4a
*Intracoronary thrombus
distal to stenosis in the
RCA. Temporary pacing wire
also in situ.*

ranges widely, from as little as 1% in early retrospective studies[32] to 52% in more recent prospective studies.[33] Although some degree of variation could be explained by differences in the definition of unstable angina, the patient population, the type of study and the angiographic appearance of intracoronary thrombus, certain factors have emerged as being associated with its presence. Intracoronary thrombus has been observed more frequently within the unstable angina group in patients with rest and crescendo angina compared to those with new-onset angina.[24] Although its angiographic detection may be related to factors such as whether or not the patient was on heparin prior to catheterization, it is now known that a major determinant of its identification is the timing of angiography in relation to the last episode of angina. Angiographically evident thrombi are particularly common in patients studied within hours of a rest angina attack. Freeman et al in their prospective study showed that the important temporal link was between the presence of chest pain and intracoronary thrombus rather than the timing of angiography after admission. Seventy-eight patients with unstable angina were randomized to coronary angiography on day 1 or later during their hospital admission.

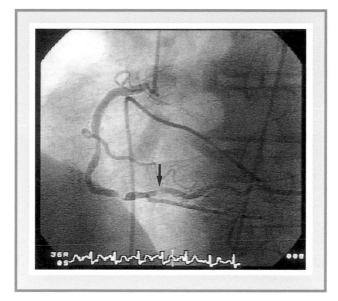

Figure 3.4b
The thrombus (arrow) embolized distally during the course of the arteriographic study.

Intracoronary thrombi were present in 43% of patients who had early angiography compared with 38% in the late group. However, there was an incidence of 75% among the patients requiring urgent angiography within the late group due to continuing pain in spite of maximal medical treatment. Overall, the frequency of coronary thrombus was 50% in patients who had angiography within 24 h of rest pain.[20] Capone et al similarly found that the frequency of coronary thrombi was 52% if angiography was performed within 24 h of symptoms, compared with 28% in patients with angiography performed 1–14 days after rest pain.[34] Freeman et al also identified that the angiographic detection of complex or ulcerated lesions was associated with an increased likelihood of thrombosis. ST segment shift on admission ECG predicted increased frequency of coronary thrombus and complex morphology.

Unstable versus stable angina
Studies comparing patients with unstable and stable angina have found that the angiographic evidence of thrombus is much greater in unstable as opposed to stable angina (27.1% and 3.3% respectively in the series reported by Hussain et al[24]). De Feyter et al in a study using intracoronary angioscopy found

that plaque rupture and thrombosis were present in 17% of cases of stable angina compared with 68% in unstable cases.[35]

Implications of angiographic detection of intracoronary thrombus

The location and volume of thrombus may have clinical relevance when angioplasty is considered as a treatment option. Interventionists have noticed an increased incidence of acute vessel closure during angioplasty in the presence of proximal or distal thrombi.[7] Intracoronary thrombi have the potential to embolize downstream and may result in microinfarcts. Falk studied epicardial arteries and myocardium microscopically in 25 cases of sudden death due to acute coronary thrombosis. Eighty-one per cent of the thrombi had a layered structure with thrombus material of differing age, in keeping with repeated mural deposits over a period of time. It is of note that there was evidence of fragmentation of thrombus in 73% of cases with peripheral embolization and associated microinfarction.[23]

Detection of thrombus by coronary angiography is also an important predictive factor of subsequent adverse cardiac events. In a case control study using data from the Coronary Artery Surgery Study registry, Ellis et al studied morphological features of the left anterior descending coronary artery in 118 medically treated patients with a subsequent anterior myocardial infarction during a 3-year follow-up compared with 141 medically treated patients with no infarction. Lesion 'roughness' and length strongly predicted risk of infarction. Eccentricity, ulceration and thrombus also predicted increased risk.[36]

The study by Freeman et al, which has also been previously mentioned, aimed to look at the frequency of intracoronary thrombus and complex coronary morphology relative to the time of symptomatic presentation, and the impact of angiographic features on outcome.[20] It was an important landmark study in that it was prospective, many of the other data being retrospective and with varying timing of angiography relative to symptoms. In-hospital cardiac events including death, myocardial infarction and urgent revascularization after an episode of unstable angina were more frequent in patients with coronary thrombus (Table 3.1), complex coronary morphology and multivessel disease. However, the presence of coronary thrombus was the best angiographic predictor of cardiac events.

The risk of an adverse cardiac outcome was greatest in patients with intracoronary thrombus, followed by those with multivessel disease. This study highlights the fact that, in spite of the limitations of angiography compared with angioscopy, the angiographic detection of intracoronary thrombus has important prognostic implications.

Table 3.1
Relation between coronary thrombus and hospital events in unstable angina (adapted from Freeman et al).[20]

	Thrombus present	**No thrombus**
Death	*4 (13)*	*0 (0)*
Myocardial infarction	*6 (19)*	*0 (0)*
Urgent revascularization	*13 (41)*	*8 (17)*
Figures give number of patients (%).		

Conclusion

Qualitative assessment of coronary lesion morphology has an important role in cardiac catheterization of patients with angina. Stable and unstable angina can often be differentiated angiographically by lesion morphology. This, in addition to the angiographic presence of thrombus, has important prognostic implications and may influence management decisions.

At the beginning of this chapter, the aim of cardiac catheterization in unstable angina was outlined as providing information to help devise a management strategy for the patient. This can range from medical therapy outlined in the previous chapter to percutaneous coronary angioplasty or coronary artery bypass grafting, both of which are outlined in subsequent chapters. However, over the past few decades, as well as providing information regarding the individual patient, findings at

cardiac catheterization have also added greatly to our understanding of the pathogenesis and pathophysiology of unstable angina. However, many questions remain unanswered. Perhaps lessons learned from angiography may help in the future to achieve the fundamental goal in unstable angina, namely control of the process that leads to accelerated atherosclerosis.

References

1. Braunwald E, Mark DB, Jones RH et al, *Unstable Angina: Diagnosis and Management. Clinical Practice Guideline Number 10 (amended).* AHCPR Publication No. 94-0602. Agency for Health Care Policy and Research and the National Heart, Lung, and Blood Institute, Public Health Service, US Department of Health and Human Services; Rockville, MD, 1994.

2. TIMI IIIB investigators, Effects of tissue plasminogen activator and a comparison of early invasive and conservative strategies in unstable angina and non Q wave myocardial infarction, *Circulation* 1994; **89**: 1545–56.

3. Butman SM, Olson HG, Gardin JM et al, Submaximal exercise testing after stabilisation of angina pectoris, *J Am Coll Cardiol* 1984; 4: 667–73.

4. Gersh BJ, Braunwald E, Rutherford JD, Chronic coronary artery disease. In Braunwald E, ed., *Heart Disease. A Textbook of Cardiovascular Medicine*, 5th edn. (WB Saunders: Philadelphia, 1997) 240–72.

5. Van Miltenburg-van Zijl AJM, Simoons ML, Bossuyt PMM et al, Variation in the use of coronary angiography in patients with unstable angina is related to differences in patient population and availability of angiography facilities, without affecting prognosis, *Eur Heart J* 1996; 17: 1828–35.

6. Prinzmetal M, Kennamer R, Merliss R et al, Angina pectoris I. A variant form of angina pectoris, *Am J Med* 1959; 27: 375–88.

7. Ambrose JA, Israel DH, Angiography in unstable angina, *Am J Cardiol* 1991; 68: 78B–84B.

8. Levin DC, Fallon JT, Significance of the angiographic morphology of localised coronary stenosis. Histopathologic correlations, *Circulation* 1985; 66: 316.

9. Ambrose JA, Winters SL, Stern A et al, Angiographic morphology and pathogenesis of unstable angina pectoris, *J Am Coll Cardiol* 1985; 5: 609–16.

10. Ryan TJ, Bauman WB, Kennedy JW et al, Guidelines for percutaneous transluminal coronary angioplasty: a report of the American Heart Association/American College of Cardiology Task Force on Assessment of Diagnostic and Therapeutic Cardiovascular Procedures (Subcommittee on Percutaneous Coronary Angioplasty), *Circulation* 1993; 88: 2987.

11. Théroux P, Angiographic and clinical progression in unstable angina. From clinical observations to clinical trials, *Circulation* 1995; 91(9): 2295–8.

12. Ghazzal ZMB, Hearn J, Litvack F et al, Morphological predictors of acute complications after percutaneous excimer laser coronary angioplasty. Results of a comprehensive angiographic analysis: importance of the eccentricity index, *Circulation* 1992; 86: 820.

13. Ambrose JA, Winters SL, Arora RR et al, Angiographic evolution of coronary artery morphology in unstable angina, *J Am Coll Cardiol* 1986; 7: 472–8.

14. Bogaty P, Hackett D, Davies G, Maseri A, Vasoreactivity of the culprit lesion in unstable angina, *Circulation* 1994; 90: 5–11.

15. Wilson RF, Holida MD, White CW, Quantitative angiographic morphology of coronary stenoses leading to myocardial infarction or unstable angina, *Circulation* 1986; 73(2): 286–93.

16. Fuster V, Elucidation of the role of plaque instability and rupture in acute coronary events, *Am J Cardiol* 1995; 76: 24C–33C.

17. Moise A, Théroux P, Descoings B et al, Unstable angina and progression of coronary atherosclerosis, *N Engl J Med* 1983; 309: 685–95.

18. Williams AE, Freeman MR, Chisholm RJ et al, Angiographic morphology in unstable angina pectoris, *Am J Cardiol* 1988; 62: 1024–7.

19. Bugiardini R, Pozzati A, Borghi A et al, Angiographic morphology in unstable angina and its relation to transient myocardial ischaemia and hospital outcome, *Am J Cardiol* 1991; 67: 460–4.

20. Freeman MR, Williams AE, Chisholm RJ, Armstrong PW, Intracoronary thrombus and complex morphology in unstable angina. Relation to timing of angiography and in-hospital cardiac events, *Circulation* 1989; **80:** 17–23.

21. Kaski JC, Chester MR, Chen L, Katritsis D, Rapid angiographic progression of coronary artery disease in patients with angina pectoris, *Circulation* 1995; **92:** 2058–65.

22. Chen L, Chester MR, Redwood S et al, Angiographic stenosis progression and coronary events in patients with 'stabilized' unstable angina, *Circulation* 1995; **91:** 2319–24.

23. Falk E, Unstable angina with fatal outcome: dynamic coronary thrombosis leading to infarction and/or sudden death, *Circulation* 1985; **71:** 699–708.

24. Hussain KMA, Gould L, Bharathan T et al, Arteriographic morphology and intracoronary thrombus in patients with unstable angina, non Q wave myocardial infarction and stable angina pectoris, *Angiology* 1995; **46**(3): 181–9.

25. Bittl JA, Levin DC, Coronary arteriography. In: Braunwald E, ed. *Heart Disease. A Textbook of Cardiovascular Medicine,* 5th edn. (WB Saunders: Philadelphia, 1997) 240–72.

26. TIMI IIIA investigators: Early effects of tissue-type plasminogen activator added to conventional therapy on the culprit coronary lesion in patients presenting with ischaemia cardiac pain at rest: results of the Thrombolysis in Myocardial Ischaemia (TIMI IIIA) trial, *Circulation* 1993; **87:** 38.

27. Taeymans Y, Théroux P, Lespérance J, Waters DD, Quantitative angiographic morphology of the coronary artery lesions at risk of thrombotic occlusion, *Circulation* 1992; **85:** 78–85.

28. Mizuno K, Satomura K, Miyamoto A et al, Angioscopic evaluation of coronary artery thrombi in acute coronary syndromes, *N Engl J Med* 1992; **326:** 287–91.

29. Gotoh K, Minamino T, Katoh O et al, The role of intracoronary thrombus in unstable angina: angiographic assessment and thrombolytic therapy during ongoing anginal attacks, *Circulation* 1988; **77**(3): 526–34.

30. Pandian NG, Kreis A, Brockway B, Detection of intraarterial thrombus by intravascular high frequency two-dimensional ultrasound imaging in vitro and in vivo studies, *Am J Cardiol* 1990; **65:** 1280.

31. Lee DY, Eigler N, Fishbein MC et al, Identification of intracoronary thrombus and demonstration of thrombectomy by intravascular ultrasound imaging, *Am J Cardiol* 1994; **73:** 522.

32. Holmes DR Jr, Hartzler GO, Smith HG, Fuster V, Coronary artery thrombosis in patients with unstable angina, *Br Heart J* 1981; **45:** 411–16.

33. Suryapranata H, de Feyter PJ, Serruys PW, Coronary angioplasty in patients with unstable angina pectoris: is there a role for thrombolysis? *J Am Coll Cardiol* 1988; **12**(suppl A): 69A–77A.

34. Capone G, Wolf NM, Meyer B, Meister SG, Frequency of intracoronary filling defects by angiography in angina pectoris at rest, *Am J Cardiol* 1985; **56:** 403–6.

35. De Feyter PJ, Ozaki Y, Baptista J et al, Ischaemia-related lesion characteristics in patients with stable or unstable angina, *Circulation* 1995; **92:** 1408–13.

36. Ellis S, Alderman EI, Cain K et al, Morphology of left anterior descending coronary territory lesions as a predictor of anterior myocardial infarction: a CASS registry study, *J Am Coll Cardiol* 1989; **13:** 1481–91.

Coronary angioplasty

James A Hall

4

Introduction

Percutaneous coronary angioplasty (PTCA) was first reported as a treatment for unstable angina in 1981.[1] Although unstable angina was initially considered a relative contraindication to PTCA, it has rapidly become one of the commonest clinical conditions requiring the attention of an interventional cardiologist.[2]

Since 1981, treatment strategies have evolved considerably. There have been improvements in drug therapies, improvements in PTCA techniques (including adjunctive drug therapies and new devices) and improvements in the tailoring of treatments and interventions to individuals at different levels of risk.

PTCA for the treatment of unstable angina is a double-edged sword, since it has the potential to worsen plaque disruption. This can trigger greater platelet adhesion, thrombus formation and vasoconstriction with resultant decreased coronary flow and worsening ischaemia. On the other hand, by dispersing thrombus, compressing plaque and stretching the vessel wall, coronary flow can be increased to relieve ischaemia. In considering PTCA for patients with unstable angina, the evidence has to be sifted to answer the basic questions of which patients need which treatments and how and when they should be applied.

Early experience of PTCA for unstable angina

Unstable angina is a serious medical condition the outcome of which may be myocardial infarction (MI) and death. Patients may also develop limiting angina and recurrent ischaemia, or occasionally the episode may resolve without sequelae.

Prior to the introduction of PTCA, the outcome for patients admitted to hospital with unstable angina was, by 6 months, a mortality of around 7% and a MI rate of around 10%.[3] Intervention with angioplasty aimed to improve these outcomes but it was apparent at an early stage that PTCA for unstable angina could be associated with a high complication rate. Even when used for the treatment of stable angina, PTCA-induced plaque disruption with platelet adhesion, thrombus formation, and vasoconstriction can lead to threatened or actual vessel closure, producing a clinical syndrome akin to unstable angina. Acute vessel closure (and its sequelae) complicating PTCA is commoner in

unstable angina.[3] One early series reported an in-hospital mortality of 5.4% and MI rate of 7.7%, admittedly in a high-risk cohort with 'refractory unstable angina'.[4]

PTCA for unstable angina—the underlying 'hot lesion'

Pathological studies have indicated that the coronary lesion being treated in unstable angina, the acute plaque event with plaque disruption and intracoronary thrombus, is very different from that in stable angina.[5]

Coronary angiography may demonstrate globular intraluminal filling defects in patients with unstable angina. In the TIMI IIIA study, such 'definite thrombi' were detected in 17% of patients.[6] Other angiographic findings, such as lesion haziness, considered to be indicators of 'probable thrombi', were found in 40% of patients. However, the precise proportion of patients with these findings varies greatly between studies, depending on case mix (e.g. the inclusion or exclusion of non-Q-wave MI patients), the timing of angiography (e.g. within 24 h of presentation versus after several days of 'stabilization') and the intensity of pre-angiography antithrombotic treatment. For example, in a study of Hirulog, angiographic thrombus (vessel occlusion or intracoronary filling defect or lesion haziness with ulceration) was found in only 14% of patients.[7] Intravascular ultrasound (IVUS) shows appearances consistent with mural or intraluminal thrombus in 78% of unstable patients, but in only 7% of patients with stable angina. The lesions in unstable angina also differ by being more likely to contain echolucent zones which may represent the presence of lipid pools (72% of unstable lesions compared with 47% of stable lesions).[8] Coronary atherectomy specimens from patients with unstable angina have detected thrombus in 35% of patients.[9] Interestingly, this study also found thrombus in 17% of patients with stable angina. It is unclear whether this was fresh or old and it may be an indication of the role of thrombus incorporation within vessel walls as a mechanism of lesion growth.[4]

Coronary angioscopy is more sensitive than other techniques for assessing the morphology of the coronary lesions in unstable angina, since it involves direct visualization of the lumen and vessel surface. Angioscopy has shown intracoronary thrombus in most patients with unstable angina, 90% and 74%.[10,11] Angiography has a sensitivity of only 27% for the detection of intracoronary thrombus, with a specificity of 92%; some intraluminal filling defects are not thrombus but disrupted atheromatous plaque.[11] In patients with unstable angina post-MI (treated with thrombolysis), angioscopy shows

intracoronary thrombus in 100% (only 35% detectable angiographically) compared with only 15% of matched post-MI patients without angina.[12] There is a very low incidence of thrombus in patients undergoing angioscopy prior to PTCA for stable angina (<5%). There are other important and consistently reported features of coronary lesions associated with unstable angina.[10–15] Occlusive thrombi are rare, unlike in acute MI, where studies show 100% occlusive thrombi unless there is pretreatment with thrombolysis. The thrombi are white (platelet-rich) or mixed white and red, unlike in MI, where they are predominantly red. The plaque is often found to be ulcerated or disrupted. The underlying plaque is usually yellow; this is assumed to be because it is lipid-rich with lipid pools (similar to IVUS echolucent zones?) and with a non-fibrotic thin cap.

The enhanced specificity of angioscopy makes it a better predictor of complications of PTCA. The presence of adverse angioscopic findings (disrupted yellow plaque with or without thrombus) predicts an eight-fold increase in risk of acute occlusion, MI or need for emergency coronary artery bypass graft (CABG) following PTCA.[13] Angioscopy has also shown that prior thrombolytic treatment for MI does not remove all thrombus and worsens plaque ulceration/complexity.[15] Serial angioscopic studies in MI suggest that the features of an acute plaque event (intracoronary or mural thrombus with a yellow disrupted plaque) persist for at least 1 month, with resolution seen after 2 months.[10,15]

The acute plaque event is also accompanied by an inflammatory response. Locally within the plaque, there is an inflammatory cell infiltrate, as illustrated by atherectomy specimens showing inflammation in 52% of unstable lesions, but only 6% of stable lesions.[9] There is also a systemic inflammatory response with raised plasma markers of inflammation. The level of inflammatory response corresponds to the clinical grading of instability and is a marker of prognosis.[16] The inflammatory response does not appear to be a reaction to ischaemia.[17] PTCA-induced plaque disruption in a lesion underlying stable angina does not lead to raised plasma inflammatory markers. However, PTCA-induced plaque disruption of a lesion underlying unstable angina does accentuate the systemic rise in inflammatory markers, and the degree of rise is a predictor of restenosis.[18] Currently used antiplatelet regimens may influence the inflammatory response.[19] However, there are still many unanswered questions relating to this interesting avenue of research, and it is unclear what benefits may accrue from modification of the inflammatory component and how it might be achieved.

These various methods of studying the coronary lesions of unstable angina produce an overall picture of the 'hot lesion'. Intracoronary thrombus is more likely to be present than not, and the interventional cardiologist should assume that thrombus is present in all unstable lesions, whether visible angiographically or not. When it is visible angiographically, it probably represents a particularly high thrombus burden rather than a distinct clinical entity. The underlying plaque is usually disrupted prior to intervention and is a vulnerable plaque with lipid pools and ongoing inflammation. The unstable plaque takes time to heal and change from the yellow plaque with ulceration/complexity to a white plaque. These features of the 'hot lesion' of unstable angina probably account for the increased complications of PTCA in the setting of unstable angina. The timing of the process of resolution of the 'hot lesion' is uncertain. How resolution is altered by treatments and which are the most important components as regards avoidance of adverse clinical events are as yet only imperfectly understood.

How to deal with the 'hot lesion'—avoidance (a cooling off period)

One way to avoid the complications of PTCA in unstable angina is not to undertake PTCA. Retrospective single-centre studies have defined various 'vulnerable periods', with the suggestion that delay of PTCA beyond a certain time allows PTCA to be performed with the same safety as in patients with stable angina. Rozenmann et al found that the acute success and complication rates were the same for stable angina patients and unstable angina patients who were able to have PTCA delayed by 5 days.[20] Myler et al found that patients with unstable angina who could wait more than 2 weeks had complication rates not significantly different from those having PTCA for stable angina.[21] However, Antoniucci et al detected no difference in acute ischaemic complications between patients requiring early intervention (because of failed medical therapy—mean 12 h and those undergoing delayed intervention (3–7 days—mean 79 h).[22]

None of these studies involve randomization, and they have varying definitions of unstable angina and varying definitions of complications. They also have low complication rates, limiting the statistical power to detect differences between the selected subgroups. They do not address the problem of any adverse effects of delay. Hence, these observations still leave uncertainty about the optimal timing of PTCA in patients with unstable angina, and it is probable that there is a gradient of risk which decays gradually over several weeks.

Attacking the thrombus
Antithrombin treatment with heparin

Heparin, in conjunction with antithrombin III, inactivates thrombin and activated factor X. Some authors have suggested that the 'standard' doses of heparin used in PTCA are too low. Nairns et al studied 62 cases of acute closure and selected 124 matched controls from 1290 patients undergoing PTCA at their institution. They found that those with acute closure had a lower activated clotting time (ACT) at 350 s than the controls with no acute closure ACT 380 s. They could not detect an ACT threshold for acute closure and therefore suggest a target ACT of >400–500 s.[23] However, this was a non-randomized, retrospective study with imperfect matching (the non-closure group had a significantly greater incidence of heparin pretreatment). This interesting question could probably only be answered by a large, prospective, randomized study of varying degrees of heparinization at the time of intervention. Such a study has been superseded by the study of other approaches to thrombus prevention.

New antithrombins (Table 4.1)

Unstable angina represents a 'hypercoagulable state' both systemically and locally in the coronary artery, and heparin alone (even in

Table 4.1
Antithrombin agents.

Heparin
Low molecular weight heparins
Hirudin
Hirulog
Argotroban
Efagatran
Inogatran

very high doses) may not be a potent enough antithrombotic to prevent the acute ischaemic complications due to activation of coagulation and thrombus formation. One potential reason for the lack of efficacy of heparin may be antithrombin III (AT-III) depletion. Supplementation of AT-III at the time of PTCA in AT-III-depleted patients can reduce some of the indications of ongoing coagulation, but in a small pilot study this was not associated with reduction of complications.[24] Hirudin is a potent direct antithrombin inhibitor, which in comparison to heparin, does not need antithrombin III as a cofactor, inhibits fibrin-bound thrombin and is not inhibited by platelet factor 4. An early trial of its use in unstable angina, in a high dose and in combination with heparin, produced an excess of bleeding (particularly intracerebral haemorrhage).[25] In lower doses, when used as an alternative to heparin, a small study primarily studying restenosis found

reduced acute ischaemic complications of PTCA in unstable angina (with no change in restenosis).[26] In a larger study there was only a small trend to lower event rates with hirudin therapy, but this was not large enough to be clinically meaningful, and this study effectively established the equivalence of the two drugs for the treatment of unstable angina (at the doses used).[27]

A derivative of hirudin, bivalirudin (hirulog), has also been studied as an alternative to heparin in patients undergoing angioplasty for unstable angina. There was no significant reduction in the composite end-point of acute ischaemic complications (11.8% with heparin, 11.9% with hirulog) or combined death/MI (3.8% heparin, 3.5% hirulog). There was a reduced bleeding rate in the hirulog group but this may reflect the relatively high doses of heparin used in the heparin group (for example, men received a median bolus dose of 14 000 i.u. heparin).[7]

Overall, the new antithrombins so far tested may be marginally more effective than heparin in the prevention of acute ischaemic complications of PTCA in patients with unstable angina. It also appears they have been used at doses approaching the maximum tolerable, and any further benefit at the site of the acute lesion with higher doses would probably be accompanied by unacceptable increases in serious bleeding elsewhere.

Whether newer agents will be more successful remains to be seen.

Thrombolysis as an adjunct to PTCA

On its own as a treatment for unstable angina, thrombolysis has been found to have only transient benefit, although a small study has suggested that a more prolonged infusion may be more beneficial.[28] Others have postulated that thrombolysis should be a beneficial precursor to revascularization with PTCA.

In patients with thrombus visible at the time of angiography, intracoronary thrombolysis can be specifically targeted at the thrombus by means of intracoronary infusion catheters. Small studies have determined that this can be done with either overnight urokinase or 20 min of tissue plasminogen activator (tPA).[29,30] However, these regimens, while successful in rendering the thrombus no longer visible and allowing subsequent successful PTCA, were not without risks of severe haemorrhagic complications. In a wider patient population, the TIMI IIIa study established that systemically administered tPA could improve the angiographic appearance of 'culprit lesions' with improved flow and reduction in size and frequency of 'apparent thrombus'.[6] However, in the subsequent TIMI IIIb trial of 1473 patients (the largest of the thrombolytic trials in unstable angina), this angiographic improvement was not associated with significantly improved clinical outcome (mortality, 2.6% placebo and 2.3% tPA; MI, 4.9% placebo and 7.4% tPA), even when coupled with a high rate of revascularization.[31]

The TAUSA study investigated the benefit of intracoronary thrombolysis with urokinase at the time of PTCA in patients with unstable angina.[32,33] The hope was that high local concentrations would be more effective at removing intracoronary thrombus and not associated with increased bleeding risks. Angiographically visible thrombus was found to be reduced (18% to 13%, a non-significant difference) but acute vessel closure was found to be increased by intracoronary urokinase (4.3% to 10.2%, $p < 0.02$). There was no benefit from a higher dose used for the second half of the study. The primary end-points of combined major adverse coronary events were significantly increased by adjunctive intracoronary urokinase. The adverse effects of urokinase were, interestingly, more marked in the subset of patients with angiographically complex lesions and intracoronary thrombus.[34]

Why does thrombolysis have adverse effects on the outcome of PTCA in patients with unstable angina? From the TAUSA study, analysis of angiograms routinely performed at

15 min post-PTCA showed that thrombus appearance post-procedure, which occurred in 12% of cases, was uninfluenced by urokinase. However, the appearance of major dissections, often progressing from minor dissections, was commoner in the urokinase group (4.2%) than in the placebo group (0.9%).[33] This finding is consistent with an angioscopic study which found a higher incidence of complex plaques after thrombolysis.[15] An alternative explanation of the adverse effects of thrombolysis is the induction of platelet aggregation by thrombolysis.[35]

Overall systemic or intracoronary thrombolysis does not appear to have a role in the routine management of patients with unstable angina undergoing PTCA, despite the observed high prevalence of, and increased risk associated with, intracoronary thrombus.

Antiplatelet treatment (Table 4.2)

Aspirin has been shown to be beneficial in the prevention of acute complications of PTCA.[36] However, aspirin may not be a potent enough antiplatelet agent in the setting of unstable angina, a hypercoagulable state with evidence of platelet activation.[35]

The integrin glycoprotein IIb/IIIa (GP IIb/IIIa) receptor on the platelet surface represents the final common pathway of

Table 4.2
Antiplatelet agents.

Aspirin
Ticlopidine
Clopidogrel
Glycoprotein IIb/IIIa antagonists
    Abciximab (Reo Pro)
    Tirofiban (Aggrastat)
    Eptifibatide (Integrilin)
    Lamifiban
    Xemilofiban
    Sibrafiban
    DMP754
    Orofiban

platelet aggregation. The binding of circulating adhesive macromolecules, particularly fibrinogen and von Willebrand factor, leads to aggregation by cross-linking receptors on adjacent platelets. Profound inhibition of platelet aggregation occurs with GP IIb/IIIa receptor blockade.

In the EPIC study, abciximab (Reo Pro, c7E3, a Fab fragment of a chimeric human–mouse monoclonal IgG antibody to the GP IIb/IIIa receptor) was tested in patients undergoing 'high-risk' PTCA, including unstable angina.[37] Abciximab was given in addition to heparin either as bolus or bolus plus infusion. The bolus plus infusion produced more benefit than bolus alone. The primary end-point of combined acute ischaemic complications (death, MI, urgent revascularization, need for a stent or IABP) was prevented significantly more often by abciximab bolus plus infusion than by heparin alone (12.8% heparin, 8.3% abciximab, $p < 0.008$). Total mortality was unchanged (1.7% heparin and 1.7% abciximab) but MI was reduced (8.6% heparin and 5.2% abciximab). Angiographic analysis found that the beneficial effect of abciximab bolus plus infusion was not confined to, or even more marked in, those with angiographic evidence of intracoronary thrombus before the PTCA.[38]

In EPIC, the majority of the 'high risk' was determined by adverse morphology of the target lesions, but a prespecified subgroup analysis of the patients with unstable angina revealed remarkable findings. In the 489 patients with unstable angina, it was found that the 30-day mortality was reduced (3.2% heparin, 1.2% abciximab) and MI was reduced markedly (9% heparin, 1.8% abciximab). These benefits were maintained at 6 months (mortality, 6.6% heparin and 1.8% abciximab; MI, 11.1% heparin and 2.4% abciximab).[39]

The downside of abciximab in the EPIC study was the increase in serious bleeding, particularly related to PTCA access sites. However, the EPILOG study has shown that, by using lower doses of heparin and early sheath removal, these adverse effects can be prevented.[40] The EPILOG study of 2792 patients widened the scope of treatment with abciximab to patients with more stable coronary disease (unstable angina patients with recent rest pain were excluded). Abciximab reduced major ischaemic complications (as in EPIC) but this benefit was seen despite lower doses of heparin, which appear not to reduce the efficacy of abciximab but to reduce the bleeding complications to no more than seen with heparin alone.

CAPTURE was a study of the use of abciximab in 1265 patients with unstable angina refractory to medical therapy scheduled for PTCA.[41] The GP IIb/IIIa antagonist was started 18–24 h before PTCA. An interesting finding in this study was the benefit of abciximab in preventing MI before intervention, although the majority of the benefit occurred immediately after intervention. There was a significant reduction in acute ischaemic complications at 30 days (15.9% placebo to 11.3% abciximab), and MI (2.1% placebo to 0.6% abciximab). Disappointingly, there was a decay in the benefit of abciximab with time, with no statistically significant benefit being discernible at 6 months. This may be related to the short period of abciximab administration post-procedure compared with that employed in EPIC and EPILOG.

In the PRISM-PLUS study, the effects of

treatment with tirofiban (Aggrastat, a non-peptide competitive GP IIb/IIIa receptor antagonist) in patients with unstable angina on standard therapy including aspirin were compared to those of placebo.[42] This study recruited a large proportion of the patients with dynamic ECG changes (95%) and with non-Q-MI (45%). They had a high rate of intervention: angiography 89.8%, PTCA 30.5% and CABG 23.3%. There was an overall benefit of tirofiban when used with heparin (the use of tirofiban without heparin was halted early due to increased adverse effects), with a reduced composite end-point of death, MI or refractory ischaemia (17.9% heparin, 12.9% tirofiban, $p < 0.004$). This benefit persisted for up to 6 months. An analysis confined to 475 patients who had had PTCA (non-randomized) found a 30-day reduction in death or MI (10.2% heparin, 5.9% tirofiban). In these patients, tirofiban was infused for a mean of 76 h of which 15 h were post-PTCA.

The RESTORE study particularly examined the role of GP IIb/IIIa blockade with tirofiban in patients with acute coronary syndromes undergoing PTCA. This study of a 36-h infusion found a non-significant reduction in the composite primary end-point at 30 days (12.2% placebo, 10.3% tirofiban), although greater benefit was apparent at 2 days (10.4% placebo, 7.6% tirofiban).[43] This decay in the benefit was similar to the finding in the PRISM study of tirofiban in unstable angina.[44]

The IMPACT II study examined the use of eptifibatide (Integrilin, a cyclic heptapeptide competitive GP IIb/IIIa inhibitor with a short half-life of 90–120 min) in addition to heparin in 4010 patients (38% with unstable angina) undergoing PTCA.[45] Eptifibatide, as a bolus plus infusion, was used in two doses starting immediately before and continuing for 20–24 h after PTCA. A significant reduction in the primary end-point (a composite of ischaemic cardiac complications) was seen at 2 days but this was lost by 30 days (11.4% placebo, 9.2% low dose, 9.9% high dose: non-significant differences). The benefits were not greater or more sustained in the subgroup with unstable angina. The doses used in IMPACT II produce only 30–50% inhibition of platelet aggregation, and the effect disappears quickly following discontinuation of the infusion, leading to the suggestion that in this study there may have been not enough GP IIb/IIIa inhibition for long enough.

It may be that, following PTCA, plaque disruption/endothelial denudation is a major trigger for platelet activation, and it is during and after this key phase that GP IIb/IIIa blockade exerts its major beneficial effects. Abciximab has a long pharmacodynamic half-life with demonstrable platelet inhibition for several days, whereas the peptide and peptidomimetic antagonists have short pharmacokinetic and pharmacodynamic half-lives. The available data suggest that greater benefit may accrue from more prolonged inhibition of GP IIb/IIIa receptors, particularly in patients undergoing PTCA for unstable angina and particularly in the period during and following intervention.

The possible benefits of a more prolonged period of GP IIb/IIIa antagonism have stimulated the search for a suitable oral preparation.[46–48] Sibrafiban, a prodrug converted to Ro 44–3888, a competitive peptidomimetic antagonist, has been shown to be capable of inducing similar levels of inhibition of platelet aggregability to abciximab over several days. In this short-term dose-ranging and pharmacokinetic study, the only noticeable side-effect was an increase in minor mucocutaneous bleeding.[46] Xemilofiban, a prodrug with two renally excreted active metabolites with long half-lives, was tested in patients undergoing PTCA. A case reported in the xemilofiban study sounds a note of caution. A diabetic patient with impaired renal function developed haemodynamic instability requiring emergency CABG, after which the patient developed uncontrollable bleeding and died.[47] It may turn out to be preferable to use intravenous short-half-life drugs initially and switch to the longer-acting oral compounds when the patient is more clinically stable.

Overall, the GP IIb/IIIa antagonists represent a dramatic advance in the management of patients with unstable angina. They appear to be particularly effective at reducing the acute ischaemic complications of PTCA and they are rapidly becoming standard therapy in this setting. Many questions still remain with regard to their optimum use. Are they needed for all patients? How long before and after intervention is treatment needed? What is the optimum intensity of therapy acutely and chronically? What is the optimum additional antiplatelet therapy—aspirin? ticlopidine? clopidogrel? What is the optimal additional antithrombin therapy—heparin? low molecular weight heparin? hirudin? hirulog?

Thrombus-removing devices

In addition to the pharmacological removal of intracoronary thrombus, several interventional devices for thrombus removal have been developed. The angiojet catheter has been developed to remove intracoronary thrombus, and preliminary studies have demonstrated its efficacy in cases of acute MI. Adjunctive PTCA is usually needed, and whether this device offers advantages over GP IIb/IIIa antagonists is uncertain.[49,50] The transluminal extraction catheter (TEC) is a rotating cutting and vacuum device which can extract atheroma or thrombus. The 'niche' where it is probably best used is for the extraction of atheroma from old, degenerated, saphenous vein bypass grafts, allowing PTCA and stenting with reduced risk of distal embolization. Therapeutic ultrasound can break down thrombus and restore patency in acutely occluded arteries and facilitate subsequent PTCA.[51]

Formal randomized studies of the use of these devices for interventional treatment will be difficult to design, and further information on their usefulness will probably come from high-quality observational studies.

Limitations

The main risk associated with intense antiplatelet and antithrombin treatments for unstable angina is unwanted bleeding (Fig. 4.1). Current regimens appear to be close to their limit of tolerability, as evidenced by the unacceptable bleeding rates in some studies (e.g. with hirudin in GUSTO IIa). As currently used, they will enable a number of arteries to be kept patent without the need for intervention. They may also accelerate the healing process, that is induce passivation, and reduce the period of increased risk for patients following an episode of unstable angina. However, some coronary lesions will be of such severity (small residual cross-sectional area or extensive plaque/vessel wall disruption) that no antithrombotic regimen will be able to maintain the vessel patent in the long term. Such lesions require mechanical intervention to prevent recurrent ischaemia.

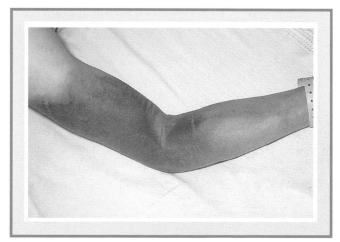

Figure 4.1
Excessive bleeding—the limitation of antithrombotic treatment for unstable angina.

Dealing with plaque disruption—coronary artery stenting for unstable angina

Coronary stents have been a major advance in PTCA, leading to reduced acute complications and reduced restenosis. The occurrence of subacute stent thrombosis leading to acute vessel closure was a major limitation of its effectiveness, and initial results showed a high complication rate when stents were used to 'bail out' acute vessel closure in the setting of unstable angina. The development of better deployment techniques and better antiplatelet regimens have dramatically reduced this problem. Recent studies have shown no significant difference in the complication rates of stenting between stable and unstable angina, even when multiple stents are used.[52,53]

Retrospective analyses of patients in the EPIC, EPILOG and CAPTURE studies have shown that abciximab treatment coupled with stenting is associated with reduced clinical events.[54] A large prospective study, EPISTENT, examined the interaction of coronary stenting with GP IIb/IIIa blockade, and preliminary results show that in a mixed population of low- and high-risk patients, the complications of PTCA can be reduced. With PTCA and stenting, the composite end-point

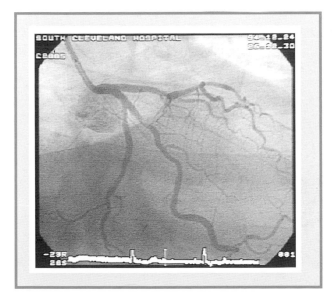

Figure 4.2
An unstable plaque with thrombus. Coronary angiogram, RAO projection, showing a large obtuse marginal branch with a proximal hazy narrowing suggestive of intracoronary thrombus.

of death or MI or urgent revascularization occurred in 10.8%; PTCA + abciximab 6.9%, but PTCA + stent + abciximab only 5.3%.[55] This study reinforces the general impression that GP IIb/IIIa inhibitors and coronary stenting are synergistic by dealing with different aspects of the 'hot lesion', stents being probably the best way of dealing with the problem posed by a disrupted vessel wall (Figs 4.2–4.6).

The most commonly used stents at present are bare metal stents, which are in themselves thrombogenic. Intense research is underway to improve on the bare metal stent. A range of experimental stents are being developed with less thrombogenic coatings, or coatings of antithrombins, or seeded with endothelial cells to accelerate passivation of the vessel wall.[56]

Restenosis after PTCA for unstable angina

Following successful PTCA, patients are at risk of subsequent restenosis and may require repeat revascularization. The lesions of unstable angina are at increased risk of restenosis.[57] Antiplatelet therapy with aspirin and dipyridamole does not reduce this.[36] Antithrombins, which in high

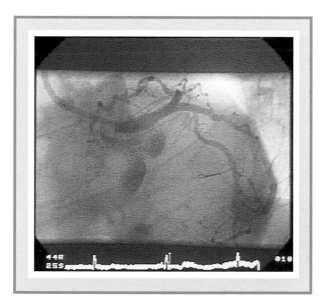

Figure 4.3
An unstable plaque with disruption. Coronary angiogram, LAO caudal projection, showing the same obtuse marginal branch as Fig. 4.2. Now the disrupted nature of the plaque is more obvious, with distortion of the vessel lumen.

concentration have demonstrable anti-smooth muscle cell proliferative activity, have been unsuccessful at reducing restenosis in clinically used doses.[26] An exciting finding of the EPIC study was a reduced long-term need for target lesion revascularization (i.e. a reduction in clinical restenosis).[58] It was hypothesized that reduction in restenosis may be due to abciximab, in addition to binding to platelet GP IIb/IIIa receptors, and binding to smooth muscle cell vitronectin receptors (α_v β_3 receptors), hence inhibiting smooth muscle cell proliferation and migration. However, the reduction of target vessel revascularization was not found in CAPTURE or EPILOG, and it

may be that the restenosis process is unaffected by short-term GP IIb/IIIa blockade. Coronary stenting has been shown to reduce restenosis in stable angina, and an analysis of unstable angina lesions in the STRESS I and II studies has shown coronary stenting to reduce restenosis in this setting also.[59]

PTCA for unstable angina—the case for selective application

Should all patients with unstable angina be treated with PTCA? The TIMI IIIb trial compared two strategies for management of

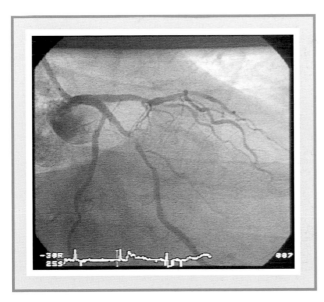

Figure 4.4
Unsatisfactory result of PTCA. Coronary angiogram, RAO projection, showing more haziness and disruption after balloon inflation.

unstable angina, 'early invasive' or 'conservative' (a 2 × 2 factorial design allowed it to compare tPA with placebo and the two management strategies). The early invasive strategy involved angiography within 48 h and revascularization by PTCA if feasible or CABG in the presence of left main stem disease or multivessel disease with impaired left ventricular function. The conservative strategy allowed angiography and revascularization for continuing ischaemia (despite medical therapy) or a strongly positive exercise test (with thallium imaging). The only benefits of the early invasive strategy that could be discerned were a reduction in hospital stay (<1 day, statistically significant but probably not clinically meaningful) and fewer readmissions with ischaemia. Mortality and MI rates were not altered. Overall 42-day mortality was 2.1% and MI rate 6.1%. However, it should be noted that the 'conservative' arm led to 58% of patients having coronary angiography, 26% PTCA and 23% CABG.[31] In a similar study of management strategies for patients with non-Q-wave MI, a routine angiography with or without revascularization strategy produced worse clinical outcomes than a 'conservative' approach which reserved angiography and revascularization for patients with demonstrable ischaemia. Again, the 'conservative' arm involved a high

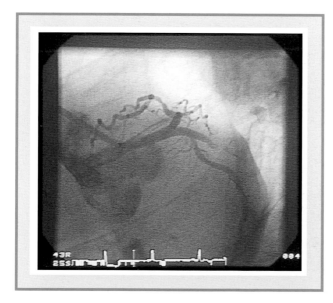

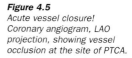

Figure 4.5
Acute vessel closure! Coronary angiogram, LAO projection, showing vessel occlusion at the site of PTCA.

intervention rate, with 48% having an early angiogram and 33% revascularization.[60]

The message coming from these studies is that not all patients need angiography and revascularization following unstable angina or non-Q-wave MI, and that targeting intervention to those at highest risk will probably produce better and more cost-beneficial outcomes. They do not indicate that intervention is not of benefit. The term 'conservative' is relative, and it should not be taken to justify the currently poor approach in the UK. A recent report shows that, despite a recurrent ischaemia rate of >40% following hospital admission with acute ischaemia or infarction, in the UK <20% of patients undergo angiography with a view to revascularization.[61]

The best way to identify those patients needing intervention is currently uncertain and the subject of many ongoing studies. Unfortunately, they will all suffer from the problems of new advances in knowledge which are not incorporated in the study design at the outset, rendering the studies outdated by the time that results are reported. Current evidence would suggest that those with refractory angina, easily inducible ischaemia, dramatic ECG changes and/or raised troponin T levels at presentation are all

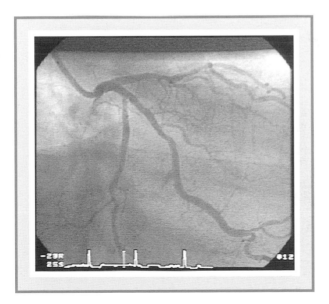

Figure 4.6
Successful stenting. Coronary angiogram, RAO projection, following insertion of a Palmaz–Schatz stent. The vessel is now patent with a good lumen and good flow. There is no residual haziness or obvious disruption.

at increased risk of complications and probably merit early angiography with a view to revascularization.

Randomized, placebo-controlled trials and high-quality observational studies help to inform our decisions concerning the management of patients with unstable angina. However, our patients are individuals, and while general guidelines can be developed from reviews of published evidence, it still requires clinical judgement to apply the lessons learned to individuals. 'Real-life' patients differ from trial patients, who by necessity are a more homogeneous, clearly definable group (often with a better prognosis). It is always wise to remember to treat patients as individuals and that trials and guidelines are aimed at aggregate populations (Fig. 4.7).

PTCA for unstable angina— practical considerations

Probably the most important aspect of a PTCA for unstable angina is the environment in which it takes place. Appropriate facilities with skilled technical and nursing support are essential. The selection of the most appropriate treatment for an individual patient requires a good working relationship between cardiologists (who may be non-invasive), interventional cardiologists, cardiac surgeons and cardiac anaesthetists. This becomes especially important in the more complicated patient with vascular disease elsewhere, for example cerebrovascular disease, where open discussion, with patients and their relatives being fully informed of the risks, benefits and limitations of intervention, can help determine optimum management. Also, even with modern pharmacological treatments and stents, some patients will require emergency CABG, and I believe that on-site surgical 'back-up' is still important.

There are a variety of strategies employed by interventionists for PTCA in patients with unstable angina. The most common is to deal with the 'culprit lesion' alone. This is usually identifiable angiographically by its hazy appearance with contrast staining of the vessel wall or intraluminal thrombus (rarely, more than one lesion may be the culprit). As well as the 'culprit' lesion, it may be appropriate to deal with other severe lesions in the same vessel. For patients with multivessel disease, the long-term prognosis is improved with more complete revascularization, and severe lesions in other vessels can be tackled with PTCA. Some operators will deal with these lesions at the same sitting in 'stabilized' patients. However, it may be more appropriate to undertake staged revascularization with emergency angioplasty for the culprit lesion and later elective PTCA or CABG. However, with patients with cardiogenic shock, aiming for the greatest

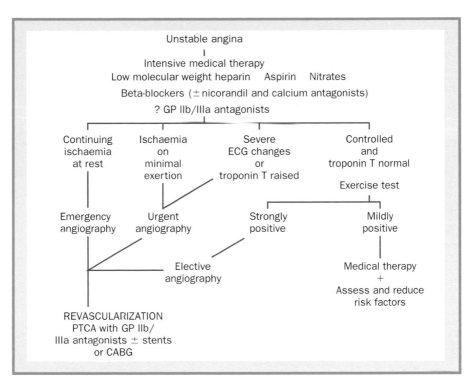

Figure 4.7
Unstable angina: proposed algorithm.

achievable revascularization at the outset may be the best strategy.

Conclusion

Coronary angioplasty has a major role in the contemporary management of patients with unstable angina. Recent developments in adjunctive pharmacology, particularly GP IIb/IIIa antagonists, and interventional devices, particularly stents, have improved the short-term and long-term success of PTCA. Such advances are, however, subsidiary to the good clinical skills required to ensure the application of available technologies at the right time to the right patients. Continuing research is needed to develop better treatments and to examine the best way to apply them.

References

1. Williams DO, Riley RS, Singh AK et al, Evaluation of the role of coronary angioplasty in patients with unstable angina pectoris, *Am Heart J* 1981; **102**: 1–9.

2. Detre K, Holubkov R, Kelsey S, Percutaneous transluminal coronary angioplasty in 1985–6 and 1977–81. The NHLBI registry, *N Engl J Med* 1988; **318**: 265–70.

3. De Feyter PJ, Serruys PW, v d Brand M, Hugenholtz PG, Percutaneous transluminal coronary angioplasty for unstable angina, *Am J Cardiol* 1991; **68**: 125B–135B.

4. Timmis AD, Griffin B, Crick JCP, Sowton E, Early percutaneous transluminal coronary angioplasty in the management of unstable angina, *Int J Cardiol* 1987; **14**: 25–31.

5. Fuster V, Badimon L, Badimon JJ, Cheesebro J, The pathogenesis of coronary artery disease and the acute coronary syndromes, *N Engl J Med* 1992; **326**: 242–50.

6. The TIMI IIIA investigators, Early effects of tissue type plasminogen activator added to conventional therapy on the culprit coronary lesion in patients presenting with ischaemic cardiac pain at rest. Results of the TIMI IIIA trial, *Circulation* 1993; **87**: 38–52.

7. Bittl JA, Strong J, Brinker JA et al, Treatment with bivalirudin (Hirulog) as compared with heparin during coronary angioplasty for unstable or post infarction angina, *N Engl J Med* 1995; **333**: 764–9.

8. Kearney P, Erbel R, Rupprecht HJ et al, Differences in the morphology of unstable and stable coronary lesions and their impact on the mechanisms of angioplasty. An in vivo study with intravascular ultrasound, *Eur Heart J* 1996; **17**: 721–30.

9. Arbustini E, deServi S, Branucci E et al, Comparison of coronary lesions obtained by direct coronary atherectomy in unstable angina, stable angina or restenosis after either atherectomy or angioplasty, *Am J Cardiol* 1995; **75**: 675–82.

10. Mizuno K, Miyamoto A, Sotomura K et al, Angioscopic coronary macromorphology in patients with acute coronary syndromes, *Lancet* 1991; **337**: 809–12.

11. White CJ, Ramee SR, Collins TJ et al, Coronary thrombi increase PTCA risk, *Circulation* 1996; **93**: 253–8.

12. Tabata H, Mizuno K, Arahawa K et al, Angioscopic identification of coronary thrombus in patients with post infarction angina, *J Am Coll Cardiol* 1995; **25**: 1282–5.

13. Waxman S, Sassower MA, Mittleman MA et al, Angioscopic predictors of early adverse outcome after coronary angioplasty in patients with unstable angina and non-Q-wave myocardial infarction, *Circulation* 1996; **93**: 2106–13.

14. Bauters C, Leblanches J-M, Renaud N et al, Morphological changes after percutaneous transluminal coronary angioplasty of unstable plaques. Insights from serial angioscopic follow up, *Eur Heart J* 1996; **17**: 554–9.

15. Van Belle E, Lablanche J-M, Bauters C et al, Coronary angioscopic findings in the infarct related vessel within one month of acute myocardial infarction. Natural history and effect of thrombolysis, *Circulation* 1998; **97**: 26–33.

16. Liuzzo A, Biasucci LM, Gallimore R et al, The prognostic value of C reactive protein and serum amyloid A protein in severe unstable angina, *N Engl J Med* 1994; **331**: 417–24.

17. Liuzzo A, Biasucci LM, Rebuzzi AG et al, Plasma protein acute phase response in

unstable angina is not induced by ischaemic injury, *Circulation* 1996; **94**: 2373–80.

18. Liuzzo A, Buffon V, Vitelli A et al, Plasma levels of interleukin 6 predict restenosis following coronary angioplasty in unstable angina, *Circulation* 1996; **94**: I330(abstract).

19. May AE, Neumann F-J, Gawaz M et al, Reduction in monocyte platelet interactions and monocyte activation in patients receiving antiplatelet therapy after coronary stent implantation, *Eur Heart J* 1997; **18**: 1913–20.

20. Rozenmann Y, Gillon D, Zelingher J et al, Importance of delaying ballon angioplasty in patients with unstable angina, *Clin Cardiol* 1996; **19**: 111–14.

21. Myler RK, Shaw RE, Stertzer SH et al, Unstable angina and coronary angioplasty, *Circulation* 1990; **82**: 88–95.

22. Antoniucci D, Santoro GM, Bolognese L, Early coronary angioplasty as compared with delayed coronary angioplasty in patients with high risk unstable angina pectoris, *Coronary Artery Dis* 1996; **7**: 75–80.

23. Nairns CR, Hillegass WB, Nelson CL et al, Relation between activated clotting time during angioplasty and abrupt closure, *Circulation* 1996; **93**: 667–71.

24. Grip L, Blomback M, Egberg N et al, Antithrombin III supplementation for patients undergoing PTCA for unstable angina pectoris. A randomized double-blind pilot study, *Eur Heart J* 1997; **18**: 443–9.

25. GUSTO IIa investigators, Randomized trial of intravenous heparin versus recombinant hirudin for acute coronary syndromes, *Circulation* 1994; **90**: 1631–7.

26. Serruys PW, Herrman J-PR, Simon R et al, A comparison of hirudin with heparin in the prevention of restenosis after coronary

angioplasty, *New Engl J Med* 1995; **353**: 757–63.

27. GUSTO IIb investigators, A comparison of recombinant hirudin with heparin for the treatment of acute coronary syndromes, *New Engl J Med* 1996; **335**: 775–82.

28. Romeo F, Rosano GM, Martuscelli E et al, Effectiveness of prolonged low dose recombinant tissue-type plasminogen activator for refractory unstable angina, *J Am Coll Cardiol* 1995; **25**: 1295–9.

29. Chapekis AT, George BS, Candela RJ, Rapid thrombus dissolution by continuous infusion of urokinase through an intracoronary perfusion wire prior to and following PTCA: results in native coronaries and patent saphenous vein grafts, *Cathet Cardiovasc Diagn* 1991; **23**: 89–92.

30. Gurbel PA, Navetta FI, Bates ER et al, Lesion-directed administration of alteplase with intracoronary heparin in patients with unstable angina and coronary thrombus undergoing angioplasty, *Cathet Cardiovasc Diagn* 1996; **37**: 382–91.

31. The TIMI IIIB investigators, Effects of tissue type plasminogen activator and a comparison of early invasive and conservative strategies in unstable angina and non Q wave myocardial. Results of the TIMI IIIB trial, *Circulation* 1994; **89**: 1545–56.

32. Ambrose JA, Almeida OD, Sharma SK et al, Angiographic evolution of intracoronary thrombus and dissection following percutaneous coronary angioplasty (The thrombolysis and angioplasty in unstable angina (TAUSA) trial), *Am J Cardiol* 1997; **79**: 559–63.

33. Ambrose JA, Almeida OD, Sharma SK et al, Adjunctive thrombolytic therapy during angioplasty for ischaemic rest angina. Results

of the TAUSA trial, *Circulation* 1994; **90:** 69–72.

34. Mehran R, Ambrose JA, Bungu RM et al, Angioplasty of complex lesions in ischaemic rest angina: results of the thrombolysis and angioplasty in unstable angina (TAUSA) trial, *J Am Coll Cardiol* 1995; **26:** 961–6.

35. Coller BS, Platelets and thrombolytic therapy, *N Engl J Med* 1990; **322:** 33–42.

36. Schwartz L, Bourassa MG, Lesperance J et al, Aspirin and dipyridamole in the prevention of restenosis after percutaneous coronary angioplasty, *N Engl J Med* 1988; **318:** 1714–19.

37. The EPIC investigators, Use of monoclonal antibody directed against the platelet glycoprotein IIb/IIIa receptor in high-risk coronary angioplasty, *N Engl J Med* 1994; **330:** 956–61.

38. Khan MM, Ellis SG, Aguirre FV et al, Does intracoronary thrombus influence the outcome of high risk PTCA? Clinical and angiographic outcomes in a large multicenter trial, *J Am Coll Cardiol* 1998; **31:** 1729–34.

39. Lincoff AM, Califf RM, Anderson KV et al, Evidence of prevention of death and myocardial infarction with platelet membrane glycoprotein IIb/IIIa receptor blockade by abciximab (c7E3 Fab) among patients with unstable angina undergoing percutaneous coronary revascularization, *J Am Coll Cardiol* 1997; **30:** 149–56.

40. The EPILOG investigators, Platelet glycoprotein IIb/IIIa receptor blockade and low dose heparin during percutaneous coronary revascularization, *N Engl J Med* 1997; **336:** 1689–96.

41. The CAPTURE investigators, Randomised placebo controlled trial of abciximab before and during coronary intervention in refractory unstable angina: the CAPTURE study, *Lancet* 1997; **349:** 1429–35.

42. The PRISM-PLUS investigators, Inhibition of the platelet GP IIa/IIIb receptor with tirofiban in unstable angina and non Q wave myocardial infarction, *N Engl J Med* 1998; **338:** 1488–97.

43. The RESTORE investigators, Effect of platelet glycoprotein IIb/IIIa blockade with tirofiban on adverse cardiac events in patients with unstable angina and acute myocardial infarction undergoing coronary angioplasty, *Circulation* 1997; **96:** 1445–63.

44. The PRISM investigators, A comparison of aspirin plus tirofiban with aspirin plus heparin for unstable angina, *N Engl J Med* 1998; **338:** 1498–505.

45. The IMPACT II investigators, Randomized control trial of effect of eptifibatide on complications of percutaneous coronary interventions IMPACT II, *Lancet* 1997; **349:** 1422–8.

46. Cannon CP, McCabe CH, Borzak S et al, Randomized trial of an oral platelet glycoprotein IIb/IIIa antagonist sibrafiban in patients after an acute coronary syndrome. Results of the TIMI 12 trial, *Circulation* 1998; **97:** 340–9.

47. Simpendorfer C, Kotthe-Marcahant K, Lowrie M et al, First chronic platelet glycoprotein IIb/IIIa integrin blockade. A randomised placebo controlled pilot study of xemlofiban in unstable angina with percutaneous coronary intervention, *Circulation* 1997; **96:** 76–81.

48. Ferguson JJ, Deedwania PC, Keriakes DJ et al, Sustained platelet GP IIb/IIIa blockade with orofiban: interim pharmacodynamic results of SOAR study, *J Am Coll Cardiol* 1998; **31:** 185A(abstract).

49. Nakagawa Y, Matsuo S, Tamura T et al, Angiojet thrombectomy catheter for acute myocardial infarction, *J Am Coll Cardiol* 1998; **31**: 236A(abstract).

50. Silva JA, Ramee SR, Kuntz R et al, Mechanical thrombectomy using the angiojet catheter in the treatment of acute myocardial infarction, *J Am Coll Cardiol* 1998; **31**: 410A(abstract).

51. Rosenchein V, Hertz I, Tenebaum-Koren E et al, Coronary ultrasound thrombolysis in acute myocardial infarction: results from the ACUTE study, *J Am Coll Cardiol* 1998; **31**: 192A(abstract).

52. Marzocchi A, Piovaccari G, Marrozzini C et al, Results of coronary stenting for unstable angina versus stable angina pectoris, *Am J Cardiol* 1997; **79**: 1314–18.

53. Chauhan A, Vu E, Ricci DR et al, Multiple coronary stenting in unstable angina: early and late clinical outcomes, *Cathet Cardiovasc Diagn* 1998; **43**: 11–16.

54. Keriakes DJ, Lincoff AM, Simoons ML et al, Complementarity of stenting and abciximab for percutaneous coronary intervention, *J Am Coll Cardiol* 1998; **31**: 54A(abstract).

55. Uren NG, Report of 9th endovascular therapy course, Paris, France, *Acute Coronary Syndr* 1998; **1**: 120.

56. Bertrand OF, Sipehia R, Mongrain R et al, Biocompatibility aspects of new stent technology, *J Am Coll Cardiol* 1998; **32**: 562–71.

57. DeGroote P, Bauters C, McFadden E et al, Local lesion related factors and restenosis after coronary angioplasty. Evidence from a quantitative angiographic study in patients with unstable angina undergoing double vessel angioplasty, *Circulation* 1995; **91**: 968–72.

58. Topol EJ, Califf RM, Weisman HF et al, Randomised trial of coronary intervention with antibody against platelet IIb/IIIa integrin for reduction of clinical restenosis: results at six months, *Lancet* 1994; **343**: 881–5.

59. Savage MP, Fischman DL, Rehmann DE et al, Coronary stenting versus balloon angioplasty for unstable angina, *J Am Coll Cardiol* 1998; **31**: 487A(abstract).

60. Boden WE, O'Rourke RA, Crawford MH et al, Outcomes in patients with acute non-Q-wave myocardial infarction randomly assigned to an invasive as compared with a conservative management strategy, *N Engl J Med* 1998; **338**: 1785–92.

61. Bowker T, Turner R, Ghandi M et al, A UK national survey of in hospital complications and management of acute myocardial ischaemia and infarction, *J Am Coll Cardiol* 1998; **31**: 393A(abstract).

Acute coronary syndromes: the role of surgery

Andrew J Ritchie

5

Introduction

Angina is derived from the Greek word *anchein* (to choke) and was first used by Heberden in 1768.[1] It is an appropriate derivation because study of the acute coronary syndrome, as it is now known, is choked with confusion. Terminology, studies in heterogeneous groups and the rapid advancement of therapies and strategies make it difficult to discern what medicine, surgery and the two in combination have to offer. In this chapter, the aim is to outline the importance of surgery and its timing, to define what it has to offer in combination with other modalities, and to outline developing strategies and interventions likely to have an impact on outcome.

Terms

Acute coronary syndrome is the latest in a number of terms which have been applied to the appreciation that myocardial infarction is frequently preceded by angina which has developed abruptly or progressed rapidly. Not all patients proceed to myocardial infarction, thus terms such as acute coronary insufficiency, coronary failure, intermediate coronary syndrome, slight coronary attack, the prodromal syndrome and acute and subacute coronary insufficiency were developed.[2] The term unstable angina has recently been used to encompass all of these definitions but it too has been somewhat self-defeating in that the one name is used to describe a spectrum of cases with wide variations in symptoms, pathology and prognosis.

This wide spectrum of clinical manifestation from stable angina to myocardial infarction includes disease processes ranging from coronary vasospasm to thrombus formation in patients with no significant artery stenoses or severe triple-vessel disease. To encompass both unstable angina and non-Q-wave myocardial infarction the term acute coronary syndrome (ACS) is now used.

The pathogenesis of acute coronary syndromes (ACS)

The management of any illness is improved immensely by the elucidation of its cause. Great progress has been made in the last decade in elucidating these factors but we still have an incomplete understanding. Angina is the clinical manifestation of an imbalance between oxygen demand and supply. Extra-cardiac or cardiac factors that lead to excess demand can make a contribution. Thus, anaemia, fever, hypoxia, tachy arrhythmias and thyrotoxicosis can present as ACS. When

extrinsic factors have been excluded, the key event in triggering the ACS is fissuring or rupture of an atheromatous plaque and the formation of a platelet-rich mural thrombus. The result of this is either partial or transient occlusion of the coronary artery compounded by embolization of the platelets into the distal myocardial vessels and coronary artery spasm. Thrombotic occlusion is the immediate cause of acute myocardial infarction in the vast majority of cases. In ACS, non-occlusive thrombus on pre-existing plaques is probably the most common cause of reduced myocardial perfusion and has been demonstrated by both angioscopy and arteriography.[3]

Treatment for this phase of the syndrome includes antithrombotic agents such as unfractionated heparin and low molecular weight heparin, and antiplatelet agents such as aspirin, ticlopadine and glycoprotein IIb/IIIa inhibitors. Where symptoms persist, dynamic obstruction of coronary arteries is likely. Essentially, dynamic obstruction responds to vasodilators such as nitrates and calcium antagonists, whereas progressive mechanical obstruction does not. Treatment of this cause of ACS consists of mechanical revascularization whose beneficial relief is directly proportional to the contribution of the organic obstruction to the ischaemia.[4]

In essence, the pathogenetic mechanisms involved in ACS are more varied than those of acute myocardial infarction. Atheromatous stenosis, altered vasomotor response, and thrombosis with or without inflammation and infection appear to be involved to a varying extent in individual patients. As it is not yet possible to identify the exact contribution of each mechanism in each individual, case treatment remains empirical. The human brain like the human heart is a large active organ with extensive functional reserve. Cell necrosis can be tolerated and the organ function maintained within certain limits. In ACS we are travelling along a path of repeated episodes of microinfarction. Once infarction has been established the prognosis deteriorates significantly. This is why 5–14% of patients with acute coronary symptoms die within 1 year of diagnosis and why the risk of death is highest during the first 30 days.[5] The challenge in ACS is therefore to achieve a resolution before infarction occurs.

Risk stratification and prognosis

Identifying the risk of doing nothing or making an intervention in all branches of medicine remains an imperfect science. It is particularly difficult to achieve in the ACS because of the heterogeneous nature of this process. However, significant advances have been made in defining and evaluating the risk for this group of patients. The classification of Braunwald[6] is based on a large diverse number of observations and the natural history of ACS from which an unstable angina risk score of 1–9 has been developed. Patients with new severe onset angina (class 1) have a better prognosis than those with rest pain (classes 2 and 3).[6] In the latter group, patients who have experienced ischaemia at rest are at higher risk than those who do not. Patients with an extrinsic cardiac cause, i.e. secondary unstable angina, have a much better prognosis once the precipitating factor has been dealt with. Patients who develop unstable angina early in the recovery from acute myocardial infarction are at high risk of developing additional myocardial damage. Prospective multivariate analysis has identified the unstable angina score to be the most important predictor of coronary lesion complexity and intracoronary thrombosis.[7] The importance of this approach and its continuous involvement is in the ability to allow us to accurately and efficaciously choose the correct intervention at the right time.

Coronary interventions — limits and potentials

Myocardial infarction or reinfarction results in an unfavourable outcome. The prevention of cell necrosis is the defining challenge of therapeutic intervention in ACS. New strategies should be aimed squarely at preventing myocardial infarction. The underlying assumption which physicians and surgeons need to address when thinking about these matters is that oxygen delivery by the arterial blood vessels is what maintains cellular oxygen. Whatever the mechanism that interferes with this, the inevitable consequence is cellular death. The basic assumption in all coronary interventions, whether by percutaneous transluminal coronary angioplasty (PTCA) or coronary artery bypass surgery, is that revascularization ultimately replenishes cellular oxygen levels. Current methods of revascularization are limited to the large epicardial arteries and do not directly affect the microvasculature. If there is disease at this level, then epicardial revascularization will not relieve the problem. Once infarction has occurred, revascularization can be deleterious, contributing to cell swelling around the infarct, thus leading to further cell death. However, the potential of revascularization to rescue hibernating or ischaemic myocardium surrounding infarcts is increasingly understood and attempts to limit the extent of infarction have been increasingly successful.[8,9] This is because ischaemic myocardial injury initiates an acute inflammatory response which can be modulated, providing an opportunity to develop significant pathways for intervention. (Such strategies which modulate thrombosis and fibrinolysis have been described elsewhere in this book.) Along with mechanical revascularization we now have the potential to restore immediate oxygen delivery to the

tissues, thus preventing further ischaemia. The current challenge is to define where, when and in what combination these can be best utilized to achieve the primary goal.

Surgical revascularization and the importance of its timing

Cardiologists and surgeons have always understood that surgical revascularization in the ACS has a higher mortality than elective coronary artery bypass grafting (CABG), despite significant advances in cardiopulmonary bypass, myocardial protection, anaesthetic and intensive care techniques. Historically, studies performed in the 1970s, such as the National Heart, Lung and Blood Institute national cooperative study group trial, demonstrated a clear survival advantage in patients with triple-vessel disease undergoing surgery versus medical therapy. This especially benefited patients with impaired left ventricular (LV) function. [10,11]

This and other studies excluded patients with left main stem stenosis, previous coronary artery surgery and patients with post-infarction unstable angina who would have been included in the modern era. Subsequent to this a number of non-randomized studies have tried to address the issue of surgical revascularization of post-infarction unstable angina patients. Lee et al investigated 1181 consecutive patients between 1992 and

1995.[12] This non-randomized study included 316 patients with recent myocardial infarction who were subdivided into four groups according to clinical severity. Mortality in the different subgroups was related to the presence or absence of myocardial infarction and LV dysfunction. Use of intra-aortic balloon pump pulsation and renal insufficiency were independent predictors of mortality.

From studies around this time on patients who were in the process of infarcting or in cardiogenic shock, outcome seemed to improve if surgery could be delayed. Thus, the timing of surgery became an important issue. Curtis et al studied 933 consecutive patients with post-infarction unstable angina undergoing CABG and divided the patients into five groups according to the time period between the initial infarction and surgery.[13] Operative mortality was shown to be least when surgery was performed 3 weeks to 3 months following the myocardial infarction and highest when it was performed immediately after the infarction.

Patients with unstable angina in the absence of myocardial infarction have previously been included in studies of post-infarction patients. This added confusion rather than clarity. A conservative approach involving mobilization, hospital discharge and out-patient follow-up, and a more aggressive management style involving early angiography and

revascularization arose. In comparing the former and latter approach, patients with unstable coronary artery disease have a much higher risk of suffering adverse events such as myocardial infarction or unstable angina (57% versus 17% for stable patients) while on routine waiting lists for PTCA. In one study, 31% of 85 patients with stabilized angina suffered a serious adverse event (one death, 25 non-fatal coronary events). Nearly 56% of clinical events were related to progression of ischaemia-related stenosis. In other words, the stabilized unstable angina patient may still harbour an unstable lesion.

In the VANQWISH trial, where the end-point was death or non-fatal myocardial infarction and which compared PTCA with surgical revascularization,[14] a poor outcome was significantly higher in the early intervention group. Of those patients undergoing coronary artery bypass surgery, the 30-day mortality was 11.6% in the early intervention group and 3.4% in the group treated conservatively in the first instance. Interestingly, 11 patients in the early intervention group were treated with PTCA and subsequent coronary artery surgery without mortality. The authors suggest that a conservative approach may be safer than an early intervention strategy. The TIMI IIIB (Thrombolysis in Myocardial Infarction) trial randomized 1473 patients.[15] Early invasive versus conservative treatment was studied, the combined incidence of death, myocardial infarction or recurrent pain at 6 weeks as the end points were similar (16.2 versus 18.1%). In the early intervention group, angiography was performed in 262 patients, for whom revascularization was not thought to be appropriate. Factors predictive of adverse outcome following an unstable episode include patients less than 70 years old, persisting ST changes, elevated biochemical markers (creatinine kinase isoforms and troponins) and recent myocardial infarction (21).

Summarizing these studies, it would appear that immediate revascularization did not appear appropriate in patients who were stabilized on acute medial therapy, whereas a more aggressive regime was of benefit in those patients who remained unstable, ie angiography and revascularization. A closer analysis indicates that heterogeneous populations of patients have been included in the study groups with small numbers in subgroups under study.

Prior to the introduction of PTCA/stenting, CABG resulted in longer survival and better quality of life in patients with multivessel disease compared to medical treatment alone. Studies in the last decade indicate that the major recovery component in patients undergoing CABG is due to the local and systemic effect of cardiopulmonary bypass.

Such adverse effects include haematologic, metabolic, cardiac and cognitive dysfunction. While much has been done to limit these effects, the introduction of PTCA was seen as a way of avoiding them altogether. However, the BARI trial has also demonstrated a reintervention rate of 42% in its PTCA group as opposed to only 3% in the CABG group.[16] In addition, 31% of patients initially undergoing PTCA ultimately underwent CABG. Clearly, surgery still has a major role to play, particularly in patients with multivessel disease and those with main stem disease (see Table 5.1), yet the invasive, expensive and time-consuming nature of the operation seem unattractive to physician and surgeon alike.

Revascularization — PTCA/stenting or surgery?

Several randomized trials have been undertaken to compare outcomes from surgical and non-surgical techniques. At least four of these studies have included patients with unstable angina, yet no study to date has demonstrated any mortality difference between surgery and PTCA in the overall group of patients studied or in patients with ACS. The BARI trial did demonstrate a clear mortality advantage for diabetics on hyperglycaemic therapy at 5 years (19.5 versus 34.5% mortality in the PTCA group).[17] For diabetics this has clear implications in the way

Table 5.1
Randomized trials comparing CABS with PTCA.

Study	BARI	RITA	EAST	ERACI
Number	1829	1011	392	127
Period	1988–1991	1988–1991	1987–1990	1988–1990
Unstable	70	59	60	83
Surgery (%)	10.7	1.2	2.1	4.7
PTCA (%)	13.7	1.8	3.5	4.8
Repeat procedures				
Surgery (%)	8	5	22	3
PTCA (%)	54	30	41	32

A lower mortality was seen in treated diabetic patients randomized to surgery (19.4% versus 34.5% in PTCA group).

Five year mortality. All other rates are at 1 year follow-up.

they should be managed. The most striking findings alluded to by these studies was in the completeness of revascularization and the instance of restenosis after PTCA.[18] In the East and ERACI trials complete revascularization was achieved in only 75 and 51% of patients undergoing PTCA, as compared with 99 and 88% in the surgical group respectively.[19,20] What has become clear in previous chapters is that the greatest limitation of PTCA is the restenosis rate and that restenosis after stenting remains an issue which is unresolved.

The belief that ruptured plaques heal rapidly and settle down after myocardial infarction is not supported by the clinical data. Around 30% of infarct-related arteries opened by thrombolytic therapy will reocclude within 3 months and restenosis and reocclusion remain significant problems in infarct-related arteries treated by angioplasty ± stenting.[21] For cardiologists the important findings from such studies is that symptoms are an unreliable guide to plaque behaviour.

The selection of patients for surgery, whether they have one-, two- or three-vessel disease, should be guided by this information. It is also known that coronary artery patency is not the only criteria for myocardial reperfusion. Other factors, like post-ischaemic oedema, microvascular injury and oxygen-free radical damage, can also limit reperfusion. The respective advantages and disadvantages of various treatment strategies remain essentially unknown. Aggressive medical treatment as an adjunct to revascularization, aimed at preventing the vessel closure associated with the presence of thrombus, is the subject of Chapter 2 and is an area of ongoing research, as is the use of high-dose statins in an attempt to stabilize the atheromatous plaque. Until this data is available, patients are guided by physician bias. Percutaneous intervention, which targets the so-called culprit lesion, and bypass surgery, which targets complete revascularization, demonstrate this 'chicken-and-egg' approach. The surgeon will often tell you that those patients rescued for failure of PTCA often have multiple vessel surgical revascularization. We do know that complete revascularization is an important predictor of successful outcome.

Reliable data comparing the respective merits of bypass surgery and PTCA/stenting in patients with multivessel disease remains equivocal. The search for the optimal angiographic result has significantly reduced the previously reported high failure rates of early non-surgical interventions. Equally, a new era in bypass surgery has also opened. We are evolving a system in which the best treatment is

the one in which initial medical therapy is tailored to risk with rapid progression to invasive management, whether by PTCA or surgery, for each individual patient.

Surgical revascularization and its outcome

In the modern era, elective CABG surgery can be routinely performed with minimal morbidity and mortality ranging from 1 to 3%. Excellent long-term benefit is related to control of risk factors and graft patency is so far unmatched and unattainable by any other method. Advances in patient monitoring, anaesthesia, intensive care therapy, myocardial protection techniques, bypass technology, surgical performance and conduit performance have contributed to the outcome. Paradoxically, over the last 5–10 years the trend has been for increasing mortality from the procedure and longer intensive care and in-hospital stay. Why might this be so?

Increasingly, advances in surgical performance allow older patients with poorer ventricular function and more severe disease to be successfully operated upon.[22] At the same time, surgeons are seeing fewer single- and double-vessel disease patients who are being managed by PTCA/stenting. When restenosis occurs in this group they inevitably enter surgical revascularization as a higher-risk case than would otherwise have been the case. The loss of very low-risk cases and the addition of the higher-risk cases to surgical case mix has resulted in a recent increase in overall mortality but an improvement in patient outcome when risk stratification is taken into account. Surgical studies have focused on identifying factors associated directly with outcome. These factors have been incorporated into risk stratification scores such as Parsonnet and Euroscore but they remain imperfect tools. Despite this, improvements in surgical outcomes have been achieved in ACS patients.[23]

The use of blood-based cardioplegia has been shown to reduce morbidity and mortality in patients undergoing urgent bypass surgery. Advances in cardioplegic protocol such as warm blood cardioplegic induction, multidose cold cardioplegia for maintenance and controlled reperfusion has been shown by some to improve mortality in patients with ACS.[24]

The use of internal mammary artery as a conduit in emergency situations is not uniformly accepted and many surgeons operating on poor LV function patients would choose to use saphenous vein graft. Spasm in arterial conduits can have a detrimental effect on outcome, although this has never been shown in a controlled randomized clinical setting. The most recent studies have shown

that the use of arterial conduits can be associated with excellent outcome in the short term, with the added potential advantage of conduit longevity. Non-use of internal mammary artery has been shown to be a predictor of increased operative mortality and low cardiac output state in one study.[25] Increasingly, it has become clear that the use of the internal mammary artery and other arterial conduits may have advantages in the short and long term for this group of patients.

More liberal use of the intra-aortic balloon counter pulsation to stabilize patients before surgery may have contributed to better surgical outcomes but has never been shown in a controlled study. Treatment of ACS in the elderly population has achieved a great deal of attention recently, as this becomes an issue with increasingly older patients presenting to clinicians. Recent studies have shown improved long-term outcome following coronary artery bypass surgery compared to patients undergoing PTCA. A prospective multicentre randomized trial (Awesome) of coronary artery bypass surgery and PTCA, which includes patients over 70, is currently underway.

New surgical directions and how they might impact

Minimally invasive coronary artery surgery (MICAB)

It is well to remember that CABG and PTCA when first introduced were controversial procedures. Minimally invasive coronary artery bypass grafting (MICAB) has developed as a method to offer the advantages of surgical revascularization in combination with the reduced invasiveness of percutaneous procedures.[26] This currently involves patients with one- or two-vessel disease and essentially the use of the left internal mammary artery to the left anterior descending coronary artery through an anterior thoracotomy incision without arresting the heart. This avoids the risks of sternotomy and cardiopulmonary bypass. Most of the recent data has shown that MICAB is safe and can achieve graft patency comparable to the standard CABG technique.[27] The morbidity associated with the use of an anterior thoracotomy as opposed to median sternotomy is not directly comparable, with lung hernia and wound infection still a problem. Moreover, this technique is likely to be applicable to less than 10% of the overall patient population and reports of its use in ACS patients remain anecdotal.

Beating heart surgery

Performing CABG on the beating heart without the use of myocardial protection and cardiopulmonary bypass is no longer a futuristic vision and is currently being performed around the world with the use of stabilizing devices that allow the fashioning of an anastomosis on the epicardial coronary arteries.[28] Indeed, it was how the first CABG operations were performed before cardiopulmonary bypass (CPB) became routine standard technology.[29]

As improvements were made in myocardial protection techniques and CPB, the original technique was left aside. However, despite such improvements the effects of myocardial protection and CPB remain deleterious, particularly to the infarcted or reinfarcted heart, accounting in large part for the poorer outcomes in surgery for this group.

Reports in the last decade indicate that the major post-operative period requiring intensive care stay in CABG patients is due to recovery from the local and systemic effects of incomplete myocardial protection and CPB. Such adverse effects include haematologic, metabolic, pulmonary, cardiac and cognitive dysfunction. Beating heart surgery has enormous, but as yet unproven, potential to avoid these deleterious effects and will be of particular benefit in patients with ACS.

Mechanical assist devices

The use of intra-aortic balloon counter pulsation (IABP) as a technique to stabilize and rescue patients has increased rapidly in the last decade. It is essentially dependent on its ability to increase the diastolic blood pressure. Coronary arteries get most of their blood flow in diastole so this technique maintains perfusion pressure in the coronary bed and increases perfusion to ischaemic areas. In ACS, stabilizing the patient and reversal of low-output cardiac state is likely to improve surgical outcome. Despite this intuitive understanding no data has been generated in prospective randomized control clinical trials, although surgeons are increasingly more liberal in their use of this technology.

Rapid advances are being made in mechanical assist devices which augment ventricular function. Mini turbine devices can provide over 5–6 l/min of blood flow and can now be inserted with the minimum of myocardium intervention into the apex of the LV. The major advance in this technology is in the powering of the device. Right and left ventricular assist devices (VAD) have a line which comes out through the abdomen to the power device. This invariably becomes a source for the tracking of infection and limits them realizing their full potential. Difficulties with thrombosis and stroke remain a significant risk with VAD devices. The newer device may have very little

in the way of occlusive thrombus developing within it and, much more significantly, the power line has now been taken up to the mastoid process, which seems to be highly resistant to any form of infection (probably related to the well-known dual blood supply of the head). It therefore looks an extremely promising device which may rescue patients who are in cardiogenic shock, therefore allowing them to become surgical candidates for revascularization and potentially, if it becomes cheap enough and routine enough, this technology could allow the stabilization of ACS patients allowing time for other revascularization strategies to be applied. The potential of this type of technology is immense.

Total arterial revascularization

Total arterial revascularization of coronary arteries is an attractive concept in which bypass conduits which remain patent much longer than currently used saphenous veins are utilized. Total arterial revascularization can be achieved using a combination of internal mammary and other arterial conduits, such as the radial artery. All studies to date have shown that there is an increasing advantage in using these arterial conduits when compared to saphenous veins. Although the superior long-term patency of the left internal mammary artery (LIMA) as a bypass graft has been universally accepted this has never been shown in a prospective controlled clinical trial.

Increasingly, studies have shown that using arterial revascularization in the ACS not only provides the patients with short-term benefit of a lifesaving procedure but long-term freedom from recurrent angina and myocardial events such as infarction. This has also been shown to be due to the patency of the conduits. In some institutions it is now routine to use arterial conduits in the setting of ACS. Although unproven by clinical trials, using these techniques seems to be safe, efficacious and likely, in the long-term, to provide a superior operation to the routine LIMA and saphenous veins.[30]

Combination procedures

A combination of minimally invasive direct coronary artery bypass (MIDCAB) or CABG with PTCA to the other diseased vessels in patients with multivessel disease is a form of composite procedure which may benefit some patients in the future. Initial results of combining such technologies indicate that a randomized prospective clinical trial comparing this combination with the standard CABG for revascularization in multivessel diseased patients could be warranted.

Molecular biology and angiogenesis

Recent advances in molecular biological techniques are now becoming applied to the clinical field with successful angiogenesis using

infusion of virus vector-mediated factors directly into the coronary circulation.[31] What role might this have in ACS patients? It is likely to take 3–4 weeks to develop angiogenesis in this setting which would preclude use in the ACS patient. In addition, it must be used in patients who have not sustained an infarct, as there is unlikely to be beneficial angiographic response in the presence of myocardial scarring. However, with the use of intra-aortic balloon pumps and various mechanical assisting devices to maintain stability in patients with ACS, this may then become a viable technology.

Summary

The role of surgery in the ACS has been outlined. Increasingly, we need to make evidence-based clinical decisions that rely on data generated from clinical trials. Because of the pace of development in technological advances and our incomplete understanding of the pathophysiology of the ACS this is fraught with difficulty. The conductance of scientifically based clinical trials is also problematical but it is not impossible if our primary aim of the prevention of myocardial infarction in ACS patients is to be achieved.

Appropriate risk stratification will contribute to our evaluation of results and could lead to a tailored approach for individual patients. Strategies to determine the exact role and appropriate timing of surgical intervention, and the development integration and assessment of medical therapies in relation to surgery, are vital. Currently, acute medical therapy will result in resolution of ischaemia for a majority of patients.

However, continued ischaemia is an urgent indication for angiography and revascularization. The results of surgical intervention have improved immensely over the last decade and significant advances in outcome are related to appropriate timing of the intervention, appropriate utilization of adjunctive techniques and improvements in myocardial protection techniques.

Advances in surgical strategy are likely to improve outcomes in both the short and long term with the wider application of arterial conduits, beating heart surgery, assist and stabilization devices, and the development of multimodality strategies. Putting all this into the context of trial-based data remains an immense challenge.

References

1. Heberden W, Some account of a disorder of the breast, *Med Trans Roy Coll Physicians Lond* 1772; **2**: 59.

2. Wood P, Acute and subacute coronary insufficiency, *Br Med J* 1961; **i**: 1179.

3. Van Belle E, Lablonche J-M, Bauters C, Coronary angioscopic findings in the infarct related vessel within 1 month of acute myocardial infarction: Natural history and the effect of thrombolysis, *Circulation* 1998; **97**: 26–33.

4. Theroux P, Fuster V, Acute coronary syndromes unstable angina and non-Q wave myocardial infarction, *Circulation* 1998; **97**: 1195–206.

5. Fox KAA, Bosanquet N, Assessing the UK cost implications of the use of low molecular weight heparin in unstable coronary disease, *Br J Cardiol* 1998; **S**: 92–105.

6. Braunwald E, Unstable angina: a classification, *Circulation* 1989; **80**: 410–14.

7. Ahmed W, Bitti JA, Braunwald E, Relation between clinical presentation and angiographic morphology in unstable angina pectoris, *Am J Cardiol* 1988; **62**: 1024–7.

8. Cohen M, Demers C, Gurfinkel E et al, for the Efficacy and Safety of Subcutaneous Enoxaparin in Non-Q-Wave Coronary Events Study Group, A comparison of low-molecular-weight heparin with unfractioned heparin for unstable coronary artery disease, *N Engl J Med* 1997; **337**: 447–52.

9. Teoh K, Christakis G, Weisel R et al, Increase risk of urgent revascularisation, *J Thorac Cardiovasc Surg* 1987; **93**: 291–9.

10. Unstable Angina Pectoris Study Group, Unstable angina pectoris national cooperative study group to compare surgical and medical therapy: II, In-hospital experience and initial follow up results in patients with one, two and three vessel disease, *Am J Cardiol* 1978; **42**: 839–48.

11. Unstable Angina Pectoris Study Group, Unstable angina pectoris national cooperative study group to compare surgical and medical therapy: III, Results in patients with ST segment elevation during pain, *Am J Cardiol* 1980; **45**: 819–24.

12. Lee J, Murrell H, Strony J et al, Risk analysis of coronary bypass surgery after acute myocardial infarction, *Surgery* 1997; **122**: 675–81.

13. Curtis J, Walls J, Salam N et al, Impact of unstable angina on operative mortality with coronary revascularisation at varying time intervals after myocardial infarction, *J Thorac Cardiovasc Surg* 1991; **102**: 867–73.

14. Boden W, O'Rourke R, Crawford M, for the Veterans Affairs Non-Q-Wave Infarction Strategies in Hospital (VANQWISH) Trial Investigators, Outcomes in patients with acute non-Q-wave myocardial randomly assigned to an invasive as compared with a conservative management strategy, *N Engl J Med* 1998; **338**: 1785–92.

15. The TIMI IIIB Investigators, Effects of tissue plasminogen activator and a comparison of early invasive and conservative strategies in unstable angina and non-Q-wave myocardial infarction. Results of the TIMI IIIB trial, *Circulation* 1994; **89**: 1545–56.

16. The Bypass and Angioplasty Revascularisation Investigation (BARI) Investigators, Comparison of coronary bypass surgery with angioplasty in patients with multivessel disease, *N Engl J Med* 1996; **335**(4): 217–25.

17. RITA Trial Participants, Coronary angioplasty versus coronary artery bypass surgery: the Randomized Intervention Treatment of Angina (RITA) trial, *Lancet* 1993; **341**: 573–80.

18. King S, Lembo N, Weintraub W et al, A randomized trial comparing coronary angioplasty with coronary bypass surgery, *N Engl J Med* 1994; **331**: 1044–50.

19. Rodriguez A, Boullon F, Perez-Balino N et al, Argentine randomised trial of percutaneous transluminal coronary angioplasty versus coronary artery bypass surgery in multivessel disease (ERACI): in-hospital results and 1 year follow up, *J Am Coll Cardiol* 1993; **22**: 1060–7.

20. George CJ, Baim DS, Brinker JA, One year follow up of stent restenosis (STRESS 1) Study, *Am J Cardiol* 1998; **81**: 860–5.

21. Vassilikos V, Lim R, Kreidieh I et al, Myocardial revascularisation in elderly patients with refractory or unstable and advanced coronary disease, *Coron Heart Dis* 1997; **8**: 705–9.

22. Louagie Y, Jamart J, Buche M et al, Operation for unstable angina pectoris: factors influencing adverse in-hospital outcome, *Ann Thorac Surg* 1995; **59**: 1141–9.

23. Beyersdorf F, Mitrev Z, Sarai K et al, Changing patterns of patients undergoing emergency surgical revascularisation for acute coronary occlusion. Importance of myocardial protection techniques, *J Thorac Cardiovasc Surg* 1993; **106**: 137–48.

24. Fremes S, Goldman B, Weisel R et al, Recent preoperative myocardial infarction increases the risk of surgery for unstable angina, *J Cardiovasc Surg* 1991; **6**: 2–12.

25. Cohen HA, Zenati M, Conrad Smith AJ et al, Feasibility of combined percutaneous transluminal angioplasty and minimally invasive direct coronary artery bypass in patients with multivessel coronary artery disease, *Circulation* 1998; **98**: 1048–50.

26. Mack M, Damiano R, Matheny R et al, Inertia of success. A response to minimally invasive coronary bypass: a dissenting opinion, *Circulation* 1999; **99**: 1404–6.

27. Shennib H, Lee AGL, Akin J, Coronary artery bypass grafting on the beating heart, *Ann Thorac Surg* 1997; **63**: 988–92.

28. Kolessov VI, Mammary artery–coronary

artery anastomosis as a method of treatment for angina pectoris, *J Thorac Cardiovasc Surg* 1967; **54**: 535–44.

29. Waterworth PD, Arifi A, Ritchie AJ, Total arterial revascularisation in acute coronary syndrome—routine and safe outcome, *Eur J Cardiothor Surg* 1999; in press.

30. Isner JM, Cancer and atherosclerosis. The broad mandate of Angio genesis, *Circulation* 1999; **99**: 1653–5.

II Myocardial Infarction

History, examination and investigations (including pathophysiology and epidemiology)

Michael H Cave

6

Introduction

Coronary heart disease is the commonest cause of death in humans, accounting to over six million (one in eight) deaths worldwide in 1990.[1] In the same year, the United Kingdom (UK) had the second highest mortality rate from coronary heart disease in the world, around 370 deaths per 100 000 population. There has been a substantial and progressive reduction in coronary heart disease mortality in the UK during the past two decades (Fig. 6.1),[2] but coronary heart disease remains the commonest cause of death in men, and the second commonest in women, under the age of 65 years. In the UK there are about 304 000 cases of acute myocardial infarction per year. About half of these die within 1 month of infarction and 65–75% of these deaths occur prior to hospital admission.[3] Amongst survivors, morbidity and mortality due to recurrent ischaemic events, heart failure and arrhythmia are substantial. These figures emphasize the need to put in place national programmes for prevention of coronary heart disease, since many of the factors which predispose to the condition are either preventable or treatable. The major modifiable risk factors for coronary artery disease are cigarette smoking, hyperlipidaemia, diabetes mellitus, obesity,

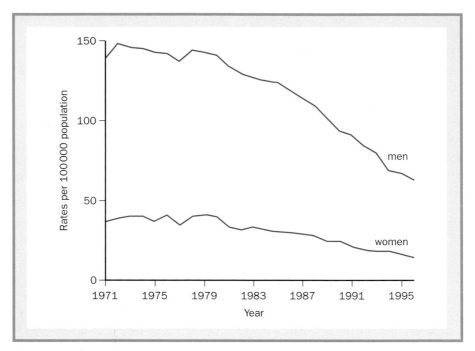

Figure 6.1
Mortality due to coronary heart disease in subjects aged < 65 years in the United Kingdom.[2]

hypertension and lack of exercise. Other important but irreversible factors are male gender and a family history of ischaemic heart disease. Numerous other factors have been implicated from epidemiologic studies which at this time are considered less important.

Pathophysiology

The initial event in the pathogenesis of acute myocardial infarction is usually instability of an atheromatous plaque in a coronary artery, with fissuring, ulceration and rupture of the fibrous cap of the plaque.[4] It is not clear why some plaques rupture and others do not. Lesions causing high-grade luminal stenosis are more likely to lead to acute myocardial infarction than less severe lesions,[5] but the majority of infarcts overall occur in relation to lesions previously causing only mild stenosis.[6] Plaque composition is important, with rupture more likely to complicate 'soft' plaques which have a high lipid content and a weak outer cap.[7] There is a clear circadian variation in the incidence of acute myocardial infarction, with a peak in the waking hours of the morning. This is associated with a rise in circulating catecholamines levels and blood pressure, producing changes in coronary tone and circumferential stress within the arterial wall which may predispose to plaque rupture. The association between acute myocardial infarction and severe stress or physical activity also supports this concept.

Following plaque fissuring and rupture, exposure of the plaque core to the circulation stimulates thrombus formation. If the thrombus is non-occlusive this may be asymptomatic, or result in unstable angina or non-Q-wave infarction. In about 90% of cases of acute transmural myocardial infarction, there is total occlusion of the infarct-related artery by thrombus at the site of an atheromatous plaque.[8] Thrombotic coronary occlusion does not invariably lead to transmural infarction, however. In dogs, coronary artery ligation causes complete transmural infarction of the ischaemic territory within about 6 h. In humans with coronary thrombosis, occlusion may develop more gradually and may be intermittent. Collateral circulation to the infarct area may slow or prevent the development of myocardial necrosis. The process of infarction may, therefore, take longer to complete than

in the dog model. In the absence of restoration of flow, the ultimate size of the infarct depends on the amount of myocardium supplied by the occluded artery, the amount of collateral blood supply available to the infarct zone and myocardial oxygen demand. Ischaemic preconditioning may also limit infarct size.[9]

Acute myocardial infarction may cause serious harm or death as a result of arrhythmia, myocardial rupture or acute severe valvular damage. In the majority of cases treated in hospital, however, the main danger is left ventricular failure due to loss of functioning myocardium. This may present early with pulmonary oedema or cardiogenic shock, or later as a result of left ventricular remodelling. Severe myocardial ischaemia causes loss of contractile function of the affected area soon after the onset of injury, which becomes permanent as necrosis develops. Slippage of necrotic myocytes may lead to expansion and thinning of the infarcted myocardium,[10] particularly following anterior infarction. These changes lead to both systolic and diastolic ventricular dysfunction. The acute increase in end-diastolic pressure leads to ventricular dilatation, which maintains cardiac output by Starling's law. At the same time, the decrease in stroke volume stimulates neuroendocrine factors (sympathetic nervous system, circulating catecholamines and the renin–angiotensin axis) which increase both

Table 6.1
The pathophysiological basis for interventions in the management of acute myocardial infarction.

Target	Intervention
Coronary atheroma	Risk factor modification
Plaque instability	Blood pressure control ?Lipid lowering
Platelet function	Antiplatelet agents
Coronary thrombosis	Antithrombin agents Thrombolytic agents
Acute myocardial ischaemia	Beta-blockers Nitrates Revascularization
Arrhythmia	Basic and advanced life-support training Beta-blockers ?Amiodarone Implantable defibrillators
Left ventricular remodelling	Angiotensin-converting enzyme inhibitors
Left ventricular failure	Angiotensin-converting enzyme inhibitors Beta-blockers

contractility and systemic vascular resistance. These changes increase left ventricular wall stress, which stimulates compensatory myocardial hypertrophy in the non-infarct zone, causing further dilatation of the infarct zone. This distorts the natural geometry of the heart and there is an insufficient increase in muscle mass to match the increase in ventricular volume. The abnormal loading conditions are, therefore perpetuated, encouraging further global ventricular dilatation. This process of ventricular remodelling begins soon after acute myocardial infarction and may continue for years afterwards. The degree of remodelling and the likelihood of heart failure is closely related to infarct size and site, occurring more often following anterior compared to inferior infarction, and is less marked if the infarct-related artery is patent.[11]

Understanding this course of events in the pathophysiology of acute myocardial infarction and its consequences provides the basis for current approaches to the management of the condition. Targets for preventative and therapeutic interventions include coronary atheroma, plaque instability, platelet function, coronary thrombosis, myocardial ischaemia, arrhythmias, left ventricular remodelling and heart failure (Table 6.1).

History

The typical symptoms of acute myocardial infarction are prolonged crushing pain across the anterior chest, often radiating into the neck and left arm, in association with sweating, nausea or dyspnoea. This syndrome is recognized not only by doctors and health-care workers, but also by many members of the public. In view of the high fatality rate from acute coronary events outside hospital[3] it should be a priority of all involved in health care to further increase public awareness of the symptoms of a 'heart attack' and the need for immediate medical help when they occur. Many patients, however, present with atypical symptoms. The chest pain may be described as sharp, dull or burning, and may be mild or severe. Patients, relatives and, not infrequently, doctors may attribute pain to 'indigestion'. The pain may not be retrosternal, but rather be located in the back, abdomen, jaw, shoulder or even in the fingers of one hand. Many patients will have a history of angina pectoris, often increasingly more

severe in the preceding days or weeks. The patient will usually recognize the pain as similar to their angina, but it may have come on at rest and is more severe and prolonged. Unlike angina, sublingual glyceryl trinitrate does not relieve the pain of acute myocardial infarction. Some patients may not complain of any pain but present with a fall, gastrointestinal symptoms, syncope, palpitations, sweating, left ventricular failure, cardiac arrest, stroke or systemic embolism. Acute myocardial infarction can occur without causing any symptoms at all, particularly in patients with diabetes mellitus or hypertension.[12]

When taking the history, it is important to note the time at which the presenting symptoms began. This is needed to determine whether thrombolytic therapy is appropriate. Certain other data from the history influence the immediate and longer-term management of the patient, including previous cardiac history, reversible risk factors for coronary artery disease, other medical history and current drug therapy.

Examination

There is no typical combination of cardiovascular signs in acute myocardial infarction, nor are there particular physical signs which are pathognomonic or even strongly suggestive of the diagnosis. As with the history, there is a classical appearance of a patient with acute myocardial infarction which is easily recognizable. The patient is distressed due to pain and fear, and may massage or clutch his or her chest. Pallor, sweating and clammy skin are characteristic features which have their origins in disturbance of the autonomic nervous system. There is, however, very great variation in the physical signs seen in acute myocardial infarction. Physical examination of the patient is not carried out in order to confirm the diagnosis (although it may reveal important signs of an alternative diagnosis such as acute aortic dissection, chest wall pain or abdominal disorders), but is essential in the early and ongoing assessment of the patient to monitor the haemodynamic condition of the patient and to detect complications.

Pyrexia is common within the first 48 h of the onset of symptoms and may cause sinus tachycardia. Other causes include pain, anxiety, heart failure or pericarditis. A rapid irregular pulse may be due to atrial fibrillation. Intermittent irregularity may represent ventricular extrasystoles, which are very common in the early phase of myocardial infarction. Second-degree heart block may be detectable as intermittent dropped beats and a very slow regular pulse suggests complete heart block. The latter may be confirmed clinically by occasional cannon waves in the jugular venous pulse and variation in the

intensity of the first heart sound. These signs may also occur in the patient with a regular tachycardia and in this event indicate ventricular tachycardia.

Early and regular assessment of the blood pressure is essential. Hypertension can occur in previously (and subsequently) normotensive patients. Hypotension may reflect hypovolaemia due to a combination of poor fluid intake, vomiting and often inappropriate use of intravenous diuretic therapy by well-meaning doctors. Transient bradycardia and hypotension due to parasympathetic nervous system activity are not uncommon in inferior infarction. The combination of hypotension, sinus tachycardia and oliguria in a patient who is not hypovolaemic is ominous, indicating cardiogenic shock due to severe left ventricular impairment. This condition is associated with cool extremities, often with clamminess and peripheral cyanosis, due to arteriolar vasoconstriction. Examination of the peripheries is important in all patients with acute myocardial infarction. Elevation of the jugular venous pressure is seen in more severe cases of left ventricular failure with pulmonary oedema and/or cardiogenic shock. A raised jugular venous pressure without pulmonary congestion is characteristic of right ventricular infarction or, more ominously, cardiac tamponade. The latter can be distinguished by positive Kussmaul's sign, pulsus paradoxus, hypotension and muffled heart sounds.

Palpation of the praecordium is often normal. Left ventricular dyskinesis may be detected as a paradoxical impulse medial to the apex beat. A fourth heart sound is common, representing forceful atrial contraction due to increased left ventricular end-diastolic pressure. A third heart sound usually reflects extensive left ventricular impairment and, unlike a fourth sound, is associated with an adverse prognosis.[13] An apical systolic murmur may occur due to ventricular dilatation or papillary muscle dysfunction causing mitral or tricuspid regurgitation. A pansystolic murmur may indicate severe mitral regurgitation due to papillary muscle rupture, or rupture of the intraventricular septum. Both are severe complications requiring urgent treatment and it can be difficult to distinguish between the two on clinical signs alone. The patient is usually very ill with hypotension, pulmonary oedema or both. The murmur may be quiet if there is severe left ventricular impairment, or loud and associated with a thrill. It is best heard at the apex and axilla in mitral regurgitation, whereas in ventricular septum rupture the murmur is loudest at the left sternal border radiating to the right sternal border.

A friction rub due to pericarditis occurs in up to 20% of patients, usually on the second or third day following the onset of symptoms. Auscultation of the chest may reveal basal inspiratory crepitations due to pulmonary oedema. Some patients with pulmonary oedema have marked expiratory wheeze rather than crepitations. An incorrect diagnosis of asthma in these circumstances might delay appropriate treatment of pulmonary oedema with potentially fatal consequences.

Investigations

Investigations are performed in patients with acute myocardial infarction for confirmation of the diagnosis, detection of reperfusion following thrombolysis, identification of complications, estimation of infarct size, assessment of left ventricular function and risk stratification. In routine clinical practice it is possible to fulfil each of these purposes using electrocardiography, chest radiology, cardiac markers and echocardiography. All of these techniques are simple, non-invasive and available in the district general hospital, where the great majority of patients are managed. In selected patients, more information may be gained using radionuclide or angiographic studies. Other imaging techniques, such as computed tomography, magnetic resonance imaging and positron emission tomography, will play an increasing role in the future but are used mainly in research at present.

Electrocardiography

The characteristic signs of acute myocardial infarction on the 12-lead surface electrocardiogram, comprising initial ST segment elevation followed by evolution of Q-waves and T-wave inversion, are well described. The presence of typical ST segment elevation, coupled with a suggestive clinical history, confirms the diagnosis and allows prompt administration of thrombolytic therapy. The distribution of leads affected on the electrocardiogram allows accurate localization of the area of necrosis. ST elevation in lead V4R is strongly suggestive of right ventricular infarction.[14] The initial electrocardiogram is diagnostic in only about 60% of cases with a final diagnosis of acute myocardial infarction, however. In some cases, ST depression, T-wave inversion or conduction abnormalities such as bundle branch block are clues to the diagnosis but are much less specific. Vectorcardiography may be more useful to confirm the diagnosis and determine the site of infarction in some of these cases.[15] The initial electrocardiogram is normal in about 15% of patients with a final diagnosis of acute myocardial infarction,[16] and repeat electrocardiograms or continuous ST segment monitoring may detect the evolution of ST elevation within the next few hours in these cases.

Continuous electrocardiographic rhythm monitoring is mandatory for at least 24 h after acute myocardial infarction because of the relatively high risk of ventricular fibrillation or other serious arrhythmia during this period.

Electrocardiography is also useful in the early phase to monitor ischaemic injury, particularly to assess the success or otherwise of thrombolytic therapy. Recanalization of the infarct-related artery with reperfusion of the infarct zone is characteristically associated with rapid resolution of ST elevation on the electrocardiogram. Rapid resolution of ST elevation to less than 50% of pretreatment levels, detected by continuous 12-lead ST segment monitoring, predicts infarct-related artery patency with high sensitivity and specificity.[17] Factors other than vessel patency, such as variation in blood flow in the infarct artery due to vasospasm, collateral circulation and the no-reflow phenomenon, may influence the severity of ischaemia within the infarct zone during the process of infarction. ST segment analysis allows fairly crude but simple monitoring of the severity of ischaemia which may be a useful guide to therapy. It is not useful in patients with left bundle branch block or paced rhythm. Continuous real-time ST segment monitoring is now commercially available using both vectorcardiography and standard 12-lead electrocardiography (Fig. 6.2).

Following recovery from acute myocardial infarction, the exercise electrocardiogram plays a major part in risk stratification and selection of patients for further invasive investigation. Exercise testing is indicated in all patients capable of performing the test in

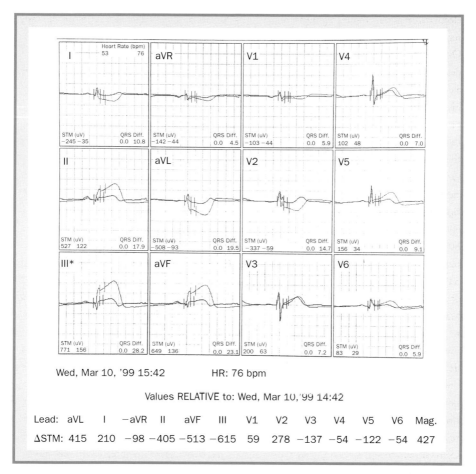

Wed, Mar 10, '99 15:42   HR: 76 bpm

Values RELATIVE to: Wed, Mar 10, '99 14:42

Lead:	aVL	I	−aVR	II	aVF	III	V1	V2	V3	V4	V5	V6	Mag.
ΔSTM:	415	210	−98	−405	−513	−615	59	278	−137	−54	−122	−54	427

Figure 6.2
Resolution of ST elevation demonstrated using 12-lead electrocardiographic monitoring (ST GUARD, Marquette Electronics Ltd). The electrocardiogram sampled 60 min after administration of intravenous streptokinase is superimposed on the electrocardiogram recorded at the onset of therapy in a patient with acute inferior myocardial infarction. ST elevation in lead III has reduced from 771 µV prior to therapy to 156 µV (21%), indicating a high likelihood of reperfusion.

whom revascularization is feasible and likely to improve prognosis in the presence of severe underlying coronary artery disease. A submaximal test carried out prior to hospital discharge or a symptom-limited test 4–6 weeks after discharge may be employed, both strategies having advantages and disadvantages.[18] Features associated with a poor prognosis include inability to complete stage 2 of a Bruce protocol due to angina, ST segment depression or dyspnoea, marked ST depression or a decrease in blood pressure during exercise.

The roles of ambulatory electrocardiography, signal-averaged electrocardiography, heart rate variability and electrophysiologic testing have all been investigated in patients with acute myocardial infarction. These techniques all allow identification of patients at high risk of complications, but their place in the evaluation of patients following acute myocardial infarction and their role in guiding therapy remains undefined.

Chest X-ray

The chest X-ray may be normal, but in cases of left ventricular failure will show evidence of pulmonary congestion or oedema. This may be delayed until several hours after the rise in left ventricular end-diastolic pressure, and the X-ray changes may persist for over 24 h after left ventricular filling pressure has returned to normal. Cardiomegaly and signs of pulmonary oedema on the initial X-ray are associated with a poor prognosis.[19]

Cardiac markers

Myocardial necrosis is invariably accompanied by release of cytosolic enzymes and contractile proteins into the circulation. Serial measurements of creatine kinase, aspartate transaminase or lactate dehydrogenase are commonly made, with a rise in serum levels to twice the upper limit of normal, confirming the diagnosis of acute myocardial infarction. Difficulties arise, however, due to lack of sensitivity and, in particular, specificity of this strategy. All of the cardiac enzymes, and their 'cardiospecific' isoenzymes, occur in non-cardiac tissues which can lead to false positive results. The peak serum cardiac enzyme level may be missed using a standard daily sampling protocol, leading to false negative results in cases with minor myocardial necrosis. These difficulties may be overcome by measuring cardiac troponins. Cardiac troponin-T and troponin-I are components of the myocardial contractile protein apparatus and are present exclusively in cardiac muscle. They are released into the serum following even minor myocardial damage and, because they are measured by immunoassay, it is possible to detect extremely small amounts in serum. Troponin-T is detectable in all cases of acute myocardial infarction within 24 h of the onset of symptoms and remains elevated for at least 5 days afterwards, and is, therefore, an extremely sensitive and specific diagnostic test.[20]

Reperfusion is associated with 'washout' of cardiac enzymes from infarcted myocardium, and serum levels rise more rapidly and reach their peak value sooner than if the infarct-related artery remains occluded. The rate of release and time to peak levels can be used to identify successful reperfusion but this approach is not sufficiently accurate or practical to provide information early enough to change patient management. Washout limits the use of cardiac enzyme levels to estimate infarct size in patients treated with thrombolysis.[21] Troponin-T levels, however, are not dependent on perfusion and can be used to estimate infarct size[22] and to assess prognosis.[23]

Echocardiography

Echocardiography is not routinely used to confirm the diagnosis of acute myocardial infarction, although severe hypokinesis or akinesis of the infarcted area is a characteristic finding which may be helpful in patients with a non-diagnostic electrocardiogram. It is, however, invaluable for rapid and non-invasive confirmation of acute complications such as acute mitral regurgitation, intraventricular septal perforation and tamponade. It is also useful for identification of right ventricular infarction, intracardiac thrombus or left ventricular aneurysm. Echocardiographic assessment of left ventricular function, by estimation of ejection fraction or using a wall motion score index, can demonstrate improvement in left ventricular function following successful thrombolysis,[24] and may be used to identify high-risk patients suitable for angiotensin-converting enzyme inhibitor therapy.[25]

Myocardial contrast echocardiography is a relatively new technique which allows accurate assessment of regional myocardial perfusion. This is currently performed by injection of microbubbles directly into the coronary circulation to differentiate between perfused and non-perfused myocardium, but it should be possible to use intravenous agents in the near future. If validated in clinical studies, this may prove to be a simple, rapid and non-invasive means of identifying successful reperfusion following thrombolysis.[26]

Nuclear cardiology

Radionuclide studies are used for infarct detection, to study myocardial perfusion and to assess left and right ventricular function. Infarct-avid tracers such as technetium-99m pyrophosphate and indium-111 antimyosin are a highly sensitive and specific means of identifying recent myocardial infarction. They

Table 6.2
Indications for coronary angiography following acute myocardial infarction.

Definite	• Contraindication to thrombolysis[a]
	• Refractory angina or ischaemia at rest
	• Effort angina resistant to medical therapy
	• Severe reversible ischaemia on non-invasive testing
	• Malignant ventricular arrhythmia > 48 h post-infarction
Debatable	• Non-invasive evidence of failed reperfusion following thrombolytic therapy[a]
	• Mild reversible ischaemia on non-invasive testing
	• Any angina
	• Moderate or severe left ventricular impairment
	• Prior to surgery for acute septal or mitral valve rupture[b]

[a]Provided there is access to a centre with expertise in angioplasty for acute myocardial infarction and no contraindication to angioplasty.

[b]Angiography is required to identify coronary arteries suitable for grafting but may fatally delay surgery in the critically ill patients.

have been used to confirm acute infarction in patients in whom the diagnosis is in doubt using standard methods, but the measurement of cardiac troponins is likely to take over this role.

Myocardial perfusion imaging, using thallium-201 or technetium-sestaMIBI, is a sensitive means of identifying acute myocardial infarction, and the size of the perfusion defect correlates with infarct size and prognosis.[27] The latter agent can be used to accurately identify reperfusion following thrombolysis,[28] although this is of limited use in common clinical practice as the scanning facilities are not readily available to the great majority of patients. In the recovery phase, there are data to indicate that myocardial perfusion imaging performed in association with exercise testing is superior to exercise testing alone in identifying patients with reversible ischaemia who are at risk of future adverse cardiac events.[29] This approach is not used routinely due to the extra cost and time involved, along with the limited availability of imaging facilities. It is appropriate, however, in patients in whom the electrocardiogram cannot be interpreted during exercise testing due to, for example, left bundle branch block or digoxin therapy. Myocardial perfusion imaging in association with intravenous dypiridamole infusion may be used as an alternative means of identifying multivessel disease and high risk in patients unable to perform an exercise test.

Radionuclide ventriculography provides a good assessment of regional and global impairment of ventricular systolic function. Left ventricular ejection fraction estimated by this means is a powerful predictor of survival, including patients treated with thrombolytic therapy.[30]

Coronary angiography

Coronary angiography is the gold standard investigation in the identification of coronary occlusion and recanalization following thrombolytic therapy. It is the only means of assessing the feasability and suitability of angioplasty or bypass grafting in patients with ongoing ischaemia, or in whom non-invasive tests have suggested a high risk of recurrent ischaemic events. The indications for coronary angiography in patients with acute myocardial infarction are shown in Table 6.2. Some of the indications are evidence based and widely accepted, while others are subject to debate, and there is wide variation in the proportion of patients subjected to angiography according to availability, regional and national trends, and whether or not the patient is managed by a cardiologist. Angiography is not an end in itself, but is performed to facilitate myocardial revascularization if the coronary anatomy is suitable. It is not indicated, therefore, for patients in whom revascularization is considered inappropriate for any reason such as other major illness or disability.

References

1. Murray CJ, Lopez AD, Mortality by cause for eight regions of the world: Global Burden of Disease Study, *Lancet* 1997; **349**: 1269–76.

2. Office for National Statistics, *Social Trends 28*: (The Stationery Office: London, 1998) 136.

3. Norris RM on behalf of the United Kingdom Heart Attack Study Collaborative Group, Fatality outside hospital from acute coronary events in three British health districts, *Br Med J* 1998; **316**: 1065–70.

4. Davies MJ, Thomas AC, Plaque fissuring— the cause of acute myocardial infarction, sudden ischaemic death and crescendo angina, *Br Heart J* 1985; **53**: 363–73.

5. Ellis S, Alderman E, Cain K et al, Morphology of left anterior descending coronary territory lesions as a predictor of anterior myocardial infarction: a CASS registry study, *J Am Coll Cardiol* 1989; **13**: 1481–91.

6. Little WC, Constantinescu M, Applegate RJ et al, Can coronary angiography predict the site of a subsequent myocardial infarction in patients with mild to moderate coronary artery disease?, *Circulation* 1988; **78**: 1157–66.

7. Davies MJ, Richardson PD, Woolf N et al, Risk of thrombosis in human atherosclerotic plaques: role of extracellular lipid, macrophage and smooth muscle content, *Br Heart J* 1993; **69**: 377–81.

8. DeWood MA, Spores J, Notske R et al,

Prevalence of total coronary occlusion during the early hours of transmural myocardial infarction, *N Engl J Med* 1980; **303**: 897–902.

9. Schwartz ER, Whyte WS, Kloner RA, Ischaemic preconditioning, *Curr Opin Cardiol* 1997; **12**: 475–81.

10. Weisman HF, Bush DE, Mannisi JA et al, Cellular mechanisms of myocardial infarct expansion, *Circulation* 1988; **78**: 186–201.

11. Jeremy RW, Hackworthy RA, Bautovich G et al, Infarct artery perfusion and changes in left ventricular volume in the month after acute myocardial infarction, *J Am Coll Cardiol* 1987; **9**: 989–95.

12. Margolis JR, Kannel WS, Feinleib M et al, Clinical features of unrecognised myocardial infarction—silent and symptomatic. Eighteen year follow-up: The Framingham Study, *Am J Cardiol* 1973; **32**: 1–7.

13. Riley CP, Russel RO Jr, Rackley CE, Left ventricular gallop sound and acute myocardial infarction, *Am Heart J* 1973; **86**: 598–602.

14. Lopez-Sendon J, Coma-Canella I, Alcasena S et al, Electrocardiographic findings in acute right ventricular infarction: sensitivity and specificity of electrocardiographic changes in right pericardial leads V4R, V3R, V1, V2 and V3, *J Am Coll Cardiol* 1985; **6**: 1273–9.

15. Chou TC et al, *Clinical Vectorcardiography*, 2nd ed: (Grune and Stratton: New York, 1974) 229.

16. McGuiness JB, Begg TB, Semple T, First electrocardiogram in recent myocardial infarction, *Br Med J* 1976; **2**: 449–51.

17. Krucoff MW, Croll MA, Pope JE et al, Continuously updated 12-lead ST-segment recovery analysis for myocardial infarct artery patency assessment and its correlation with multiple simultaneous early angiographic observations, *Am J Cardiol* 1993; **71**: 145–51.

18. Senaratne MP, Hsu LA, Rossal RE, Kappagoda CT, Exercise testing after acute myocardial infarction: relative value of the low-level predischarge and the postdischarge exercise test, *J Am Coll Cardiol* 1988; **12**: 1416–22.

19. Battler A, Karliner JS, Higgins CB et al, The initial chest X-ray in acute myocardial infarction. Prediction of early and late mortality and survival, *Circulation* 1980; **61**: 1004–9.

20. Katus HA, Remppis A, Neumann FJ et al, Diagnostic efficiency of Troponin T measurements in acute myocardial infarction, *Circulation* 1991; **83**: 902–12.

21. Blanke H, von Hardenberg D, Cohen M et al, Patterns of creatine kinase release during acute myocardial infarction after non-surgical reperfusion: comparison with conventional treatment and correlation with infarct size, *J Am Coll Cardiol* 1984; **3**: 675–80.

22. Katus HA, Diederich KW, Schwarz F et al, Influence of reperfusion on serum concentrations of cytosolic creatine kinase and structural myosin light chains in acute myocardial infarction, *Am J Cardiol* 1987; **60**: 440–8.

23. Ohman ME, Armstrong PW, Christenson RH et al, Cardiac troponin T levels for risk stratification in acute myocardial ischaemia, *N Engl J Med* 1996; **335**: 1333–41.

24. Otto CM, Stratton JR, Maynard C et al, Echocardiographic evaluation of segmental wall motion early and late after thrombolytic therapy in acute myocardial infarction; The Western Washington Tissue Plasminogen Activator Emergency Room Trial, *Am J Cardiol* 1990; **65**: 132–8.

25. Kober L, Torp-Pederson C, Carlsen J et al, An echocardiographic method for selecting high risk patients shortly after acute myocardial infarction for inclusion in multi-centre studies (as used in the TRACE study), *Eur Heart J* 1994; **15**: 1616–20.

26. Kaul S, Myocardial contrast echocardiography in acute myocardial infarction: time to test for routine clinical use, *Heart* 1998; **81**: 2–5.

27. Miller TD, Christian TF, Hopfenspirger MR et al, Infarct size after acute myocardial infarction measured by quantitative tomographic 99mTc sestamibi predicts subsequent mortality, *Circulation* 1995; **92**: 334–41.

28. Wackers FJ, Gibbons RJ, Verani MS et al, Serial quantitative planar technetium-99m-isonitrile imaging in acute myocardial infarction: efficacy for non-invasive assessment of thrombolytic therapy, *J Am Coll Cardiol* 1989; **14**: 861–73.

29. Gibson RS, Watson DD, Value of planar ^{201}Tl imaging in risk stratification of patients recovering from acute myocardial infarction, *Circulation* 1991; **84(Suppl I)**: I148–I162.

30. Zaret BL, Wackers FJ, Terrin M et al and the TIMI investigators, Does left ventricular ejection fraction following thrombolytic therapy have the same prognostic impact described in the prethrombolytic era? Results of the TIMI II trial, *J Am Coll Cardiol* 1991; **17**: 214A.

The role of aspirin, heparin and thrombolysis

Adrian D Raybould and Maurice B Buchalter

7

Introduction

Antiplatelet, antithrombotic and thrombolytic therapy have become an integral part in the management of patients with acute myocardial infarction. The pivotal role of platelets and coronary thrombosis in the pathophysiology of an acute myocardial infarction provides a rationale for their use.

The development of a myocardial infarction is characterized by acute atherosclerotic plaque rupture and the exposure of substances that promote platelet adhesion, activation and thrombin generation.[1–4] The adhesion and aggregation of platelets results in the release and activation of mediators such as thromboxane A_2, serotonin, adenosine diphosphate, platelet activating factor, thrombin, tissue factor and oxygen free radicals. The formation of coronary thrombus leads to vessel occlusion and an interruption of coronary bloodflow. This leads to an imbalance between oxygen demand and supply to the myocardium, which if severe and persistent leads to myocardial infarction. At post mortem, thrombi have been identified in the majority of patients dying of acute myocardial infarction.[5]

The routine use of therapies aimed at preventing and, indeed, reversing these pathological processes has played a significant part in the dramatic reduction seen in the short-term mortality following myocardial infarction over the past 20 years. Further, because it is a common and well-defined cause of death, larger and more sophisticated trials have been carried out which have been able to refine not only the choice of thrombolytic agent used but the overall management of acute myocardial infarction.

Aspirin

The substantive benefits of aspirin given to patients with suspected myocardial infarction were established with the publication of The Second International Study of Infarct Survival

(ISIS-2).[6] The treatment of patients with aspirin resulted in a reduction in mortality similar to that produced by thrombolytic therapy alone, and the use of both agents was found to be additive (Fig. 7.1).

In this study, 17 187 patients with suspected myocardial infarction were randomized to receive intravenous streptokinase, oral aspirin, both or neither. Patients randomized to receive aspirin received 162.5 mg/day for 1 month (with the first tablet chewed or crushed for rapid antiplatelet effect). At 1 month, the vascular mortality in the aspirin-treated group was 9.4%, compared with 11.8% in the placebo group (odds reduction: 23%, 95% CI 15–30%, $p < 0.00001$). This reduction represents the avoidance of about 25 early deaths per 1000 patients treated. There was

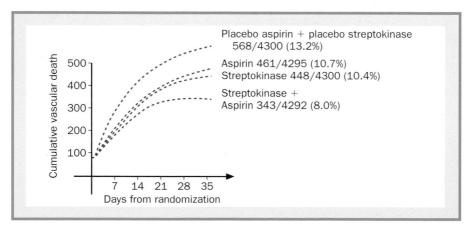

Figure 7.1
Cumulative vascular death (days 0–35) from the second International Study of Infarct Survival (ISIS2).

also a reduction in the occurrence of non-fatal reinfarction (1.0% versus 2.0%, $p < 0.00001$) and non-fatal stroke (0.3% versus 0.6%, $p < 0.02$). Further follow-up in the ISIS-2 trial showed that the benefits persisted for several years and that the continuation of aspirin therapy beyond 1 month resulted in a further 40 fewer deaths, non-fatal reinfarctions and strokes per 1000 patients treated.[7]

As already mentioned, once an atherosclerotic plaque has undergone disruption, platelets play a pivotal role in the orchestration of a prothrombotic state and the subsequent formation of thrombus. The inhibition of platelet aggregation with aspirin is now established as an early part in the management of patients with acute myocardial infarction.

Several pathways lead to platelet aggregation (Fig. 7.2). The known action of aspirin involves the inhibition of thromboxane A_2 production by inhibition of platelet cyclooxygenase. However, aspirin is only partially able to impede aggregation induced by collagen, ADP and thrombin.[8] Aspirin is therefore unable to prevent the initial layer of platelets from binding to the subendothelium or atherosclerotic plaque, and the subsequent release of platelet granules is unopposed. Aspirin is further unable to affect the action of platelet-derived growth factors on smooth muscle cells. The clinical efficacy of aspirin may therefore seem somewhat surprising.

However, there is increasing evidence that the antithrombotic effect of aspirin is not only dependent on the inhibition of platelet cyclooxygenase. For example, the acetylation of GTP proteins, thrombin receptors and prothrombin seems to inhibit thrombogenesis and is independent of cyclooxygenase activity.[9,10] The salicylate moiety of aspirin is also able to antagonize the lipoxygenase pathway of arachidonic acid metabolism in platelets, and the existence of two cyclooxygenase enzymes (COX1, COX2)[11] may further help to elucidate the antithrombotic mechanism of aspirin.

An initial dose of aspirin of at least 160 mg is required to produce complete cyclooxygenase inhibition within 1 h[12,13] and it is therefore recommended that an initial dose of 300 mg is given which can subsequently be reduced to a lower daily maintenance dose. With regard to daily maintenance dosage, studies have shown that daily doses as low as 75 mg produce complete cyclooxygenase inhibition.[14] Although other mechanisms may play an important role in the clinical benefit of aspirin, most clinical trials demonstrate a protective effect with doses in the range 75–300 mg, with higher doses showing no improved benefit but increased side-effects. Enteric formulations can be used to limit unwanted gastric irritation.

One finding from ISIS-2 was that, in contrast to thrombolysis, the clinical effectiveness of

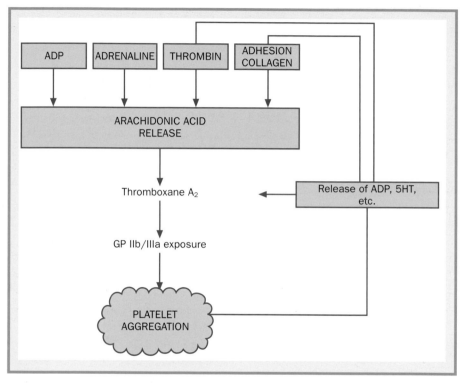

Figure 7.2
Mechanisms of platelet aggregation.

aspirin therapy is not time dependent. That is to say, patients treated 12 h after the onset of symptoms derive as much benefit as patients treated at 6 h.

In an overview of randomized trials enrolling over 20 000 patients, the Antiplatelets Trialists Collaboration reported a 25% reduction in recurrent infarction, stroke and vascular death in patients treated with prolonged aspirin therapy. Further studies have shown that patients are likely to have a smaller reinfarction and that it is more likely to be non-Q-wave in nature if they are receiving long-term aspirin therapy. As a result of such studies, it is recommended that patients should remain on aspirin therapy indefinitely following a myocardial infarction.

Despite the compelling evidence to support the use of aspirin in myocardial infarction, evidence suggests that it is still under-prescribed. In the Scandinavian Simvastatin Survival Study, for example, only 50% of patients who had suffered a previous myocardial infarction were taking aspirin in 1994. Aspirin should routinely be given in the setting of an acute myocardial infarction unless there is an absolute contraindication, such as true allergy or active bleeding peptic ulcer disease. Minor gastric irritation or a previous history of peptic ulcer disease which is currently quiescent is an inadequate reason to withhold this simple but life-saving treatment. For those with a contraindication, an alternative antiplatelet therapy such as clopidogrel should be considered.

Heparin

The precise role of heparin in the setting of acute myocardial infarction has been much more difficult to define. This has become even more difficult since the introduction of widespread thrombolytic therapy.

Pre-thrombolysis

Since the discovery of the first coumarin derivative by Link in 1943,[15] the role of anticoagulants in the management of myocardial infarction has been studied widely. However, in the pre-thrombolytic era most studies contained too few patients to demonstrate a clinical benefit which reached statistical significance. Most studies tended to favour the use of anticoagulants with trends towards lower mortality. In a review by Chalmers et al,[16] the data from 32 randomized trials between 1948 and 1977 were analysed. In these trials, 15 978 patients were examined to test the efficacy of anticoagulation in preventing the morbidity and mortality associated with acute myocardial infarction. Of these patients, 51% received either a coumarin anticoagulant or heparin or both. Rates of thromboembolism were higher in the control patients, and haemorrhagic complications in the anticoagulant-treated patients. Pooling of all randomized trials gave mean case fatality rates of 19.6% for the controls and 15.4% for the anticoagulant group, a relative reduction of 21% ($p < 0.05$). Haemorrhagic complications were two to four times greater in the anticoagulant group.

For patients who do not receive thrombolytic therapy, an overview of the available data would support the routine use of heparin in reducing the mortality and morbidity from serious complications such as reinfarction and thromboembolism.[17,18] For patients presenting with suspected acute myocardial infarction who do not fulfil ECG criteria for thrombolysis, heparin should therefore be given unless contraindicated.

Post-thrombolysis

In patients who have received thrombolysis, the evidence supporting the use of anticoagulants is less clear and the data from trials are often confusing and conflicting. Failure to achieve or maintain coronary perfusion is a major limitation of thrombolytic therapy. Thrombolytic agents have been shown to activate both platelets[19] and clotting factors.[20–22] Thus, the activation of the haemostatic mechanism by fibrinolytic agents has led to the recommendation of adjunctive thrombolytic therapy with aspirin and heparin.[23] The clinical benefits of aspirin when used as an adjunct to thrombolysis have already been established.[6] However, the clinical benefit of the addition of heparin to thrombolysis is still controversial.[24]

A subgroup analysis from 433 patients in the SCATI Trial[25] provides mortality data on the addition of heparin to thrombolysis in the absence of aspirin. In the subgroup which received streptokinase with or without subcutaneous calcium heparin, there were 10 deaths among 218 patients randomized to heparin, and 19 among 215 receiving placebo. Though showing a trend towards reduced mortality with heparin use, the clinical benefit did not reach statistical significance and, further, there were no significant differences between treatments for recurrent ischaemia or non-fatal reinfarction. Data for combined

aspirin and heparin as adjunctive therapies are available from large mortality studies with delayed subcutaneous heparin and angiographic studies utilizing intravenous heparin.

GISSI-2[26] and ISIS-3[27] are large mortality trials which have provided consistent information on the risks and benefits of combined aspirin and delayed subcutaneous heparin as adjuncts to thrombolysis. Together they provide data on over 62 000 patients.

GISSI-2 compared directly the efficacy of two thrombolytic agents, streptokinase and tissue plasminogen activator (tPA), and also tested whether there were additional benefits with delayed subcutaneous heparin when added to aspirin and thrombolysis. All 20 891 patients received 300–325 mg of aspirin daily by mouth. GISSI-2 found no difference in overall mortality between streptokinase and tPA, although streptokinase was associated with significantly fewer strokes. The addition of subcutaneous heparin had no effect on in-hospital mortality (8.5% with streptokinase versus 9.0% with tPA, $p = 0.29$) or total mortality at 35 days (9.3 versus 9.4%, $p = 0.82$). Moreover, the addition of subcutaneous heparin was associated with an increased risk of bleeding requiring transfusion.

ISIS-3 compared the efficacy of three

thrombolytic agents, streptokinase, tPA and anistreplase, and of subcutaneous heparin versus no heparin in 14 299 patients with an evolving myocardial infarction. All patients received aspirin 162 mg daily, with the first tablet chewed for rapid antiplatelet effect. Again, no difference in mortality among the different thrombolytic agents was found, although there was a significantly lower incidence of cerebral haemorrhage among patients receiving streptokinase compared with other thrombolytics. At the prespecified end-point of 35 days, there was no significant difference in the mortality among patients treated with or without heparin therapy. As in GISSI-3, the addition of delayed subcutaneous heparin was associated with a higher frequency of major non-cerebral bleeds and definite or probable cerebral haemorrhage. Reinfarction rates did not differ significantly between the aspirin alone and aspirin plus subcutaneous heparin groups.

In the GUSTO-I study,[28] no difference in 35-day mortality was seen in patients receiving streptokinase plus subcutaneous heparin (7.2%) or intravenous heparin (7.4%). However, non-randomized subgroup analysis from the LATE Trial[29] showed that in the 2821 patients who received tPA, there was a 30-day mortality of 7.6% when intravenous heparin was used, compared with 10.4% when no heparin was given. Therefore, the available evidence suggests that intravenous

heparin is of no benefit when given with streptokinase but may be beneficial when given with tPA.

In addition to patient outcome trials, a number of angiographic studies have assessed the role of heparin in establishing and maintaining infarct-related patency. In the Bleich[30] and the HART[31] studies, infarct-related patency rates were higher when heparin was added to tPA. Similarly, The European Co-operative Study Group performed angiograms at 48–120 h following tPA and still found increased patency rates among patients treated with heparin.[32]

Therefore, on the basis of the evidence available, the routine use of heparin with thrombolytics other than tPA cannot be recommended. There is no evidence of improved survival but a significant increase in haemorrhagic complications. However, certain patients who are at high risk of thromboembolic events following their myocardial infarction, for example large anterior myocardial infarctions or patients with atrial fibrillation, should be considered for anticoagulant therapy with heparin.

On the basis of data from GUSTO-I and angiographic studies, it is recommended that intravenous heparin be given when tPA is administered. This should be continued for 48 h following tPA, and some clinicians advise tapering off the infusion rather than stopping abruptly due to concern over an increase in thrombin generation and rebound ischaemia after the cessation of heparin therapy.[33]

Most clinicians usually give heparin intravenously, initially as a bolus, and then as a continuous infusion. A regimen based on body weight, that is 70 µ/kg bolus followed by 15 µ/kg per hour as an infusion, has been shown to produce a rapid therapeutic level of heparin [with a target activated partial thromboplantin time (APTT) of 1.5–2.0 times control].[34] Intravenous heparin should be continued for 48 h and then a review undertaken as to the need to continue with anticoagulant therapy based on factors such as ongoing ischaemia and subsequent risk of thromboembolism. Patients with large anterior myocardial infarctions, congestive cardiac failure or atrial fibrillation are at increased risk of thromboembolic complications, and continuing anticoagulant therapy with oral agents has been recommended with a target international normalized ratio (INR) of 2.0–3.0.[35]

Problems associated with unfractionated heparin, such as interpatient variation in terms of therapeutic response, the need for regular laboratory monitoring, inhibition by platelet factor 4 and dependence on antithrombin III, have led to the development of new antithrombotic agents. These include the direct thombin inhibitors such as hirudin and the low molecular weight heparins such as deltaparin. The low molecular weight heparins are now commonly used in the setting of unstable angina and non-Q-wave myocardial infarction but have not been studied in the setting of acute Q-wave myocardial infarction. The direct thrombin inhibitors have been studied as adjunctive therapy with thrombolysis but, overall, results of studies have been disappointing or provided conflicting results.[36,37]

To summarize, in the setting of acute myocardial infarction, evidence would support the routine use of intravenous heparin in all patients not receiving thrombolytic therapy. In those receiving thrombolysis, only those receiving tPA have evidence to justify the adjunctive use of heparin. Unfractionated or low molecular weight heparins should be considered in the management of any patient thought to be at high risk of thromboembolism, namely, large anterior myocardial infarction, atrial fibrillation or congestive cardiac failure.

Thrombolysis

Large trials would suggest that few therapeutic interventions can have had such a dramatic impact on the mortality and morbidity of a condition as thrombolysis has had on the outcome of patients treated for acute myocardial infarction. Certainly, no therapy can boast the vast number of patients randomized in placebo-controlled international multicentre trials conducted in the late 1980s and early 1990s. Such trials resulted in the randomization of over 60 000 patients to receive either placebo or thrombolysis during the first hours of an acute myocardial infarction.

The results of individual trials have demonstrated a significant reduction in mortality with the use of thrombolytics[6,38,39] and an overview of the nine largest trials has suggested the saving of approximately 35 lives per 1000 patients treated if therapy is commenced within 1 h of the onset of symptoms, reducing to 16 lives saved per 1000 treated at 7–12 h.[40] Such data have resulted in the worldwide acceptance of thrombolysis as a first-line therapy in the management of patients with acute myocardial infarction.

The rationale for the routine use of thrombolytic agents arose from the pioneering work of Reimer and his colleagues. Using a canine model, they were able to demonstrate that the amount of myocardial necrosis following coronary occlusion could be limited by the early reperfusion of the ischaemic myocardium. They subsequently demonstrated that the amount of myocardial salvage was a function of the decreasing time between occlusion and reperfusion.[41] This time relationship was not linear, however, with most of the salvage occurring when reperfusion occurred within the first few hours. Following coronary occlusion, the investigators demonstrated that myocardial cell necrosis began after approximately 15 min and proceeded as a 'wavefront' from the subendocardial to epicardial surface. Thus with early reperfusion a small subendocardial infarct results. Further studies demonstrated that the amount of myocardial salvage is also determined by the degree of collateral bloodflow in addition to the time to reperfusion.[42]

In the early 1980s, Rentrop et al[43] devised a conceptual model using the available information concerning thrombolysis. The model presumed that early thrombolysis and reperfusion results in a greater salvage of myocardium and hence better preservation of left ventricular ejection fraction. The authors postulated that the clinical benefit of thrombolysis would be dependent upon the amount of myocardium at risk from the occluded artery, the time from occlusion to reperfusion and the degree of collateral bloodflow. The predictions have subsequently been validated, and detailed studies of the dynamics of human myocardial infarction using Sestamibi imaging have demonstrated that, as in experimental animals, these factors are the apparent determinants of infarct size in humans.[44]

Throughout the 1980s, a number of angiographic studies were carried out to determine the effectiveness of thrombolytics in achieving the patency of an infarct-related artery. In order to provide standardization so that comparisons of different thrombolytic agents and regimens could be compared, a grading of flow in the infarct-related artery at 90 min was used by many investigators. The TIMI grading system was first used in the angiographic comparison of streptokinase and tPA.[45] The system scores as follows: grade 0 = complete occlusion of the infarct-related artery; grade 1 = some penetration of contrast material beyond the obstruction but no perfusion of the clinical artery bed; grade 2 = perfusion of the infarct-related artery and distal bed but delayed compared to adjacent arteries; grade 3 = perfusion of the infarct-related artery and normal perfusion of the distal bed.

A TIMI frame count, which involves counting the number of angiographic frames taken for contrast to reach the distal bed of the artery, is a means of further quantitating flow. TIMI grade 3 flow is in the range 35 ± 13 frames, compared to 88 ± 31 frames for TIMI grade 2 flow. Initially, TIMI grade 2 and 3 flow were grouped together as representing favourable outcomes; however, it is now well established that TIMI grade 3 flow is required for optimal benefit, and patients achieving grade 3 flow achieve much greater reductions in infarct size

and improved short-term[46] and long-term[47] mortality.

Coronary thrombolysis for acute myocardial infarction was used as far back as 1958;[48] however, the routine use of thrombolytic therapy in acute myocardial infarction was established following the publication of the GISSI-I trial in 1986.[38] In this large multicentre trial, 11 712 patients with suspected acute myocardial infarction were randomized to receive streptokinase 1.5 million units intravenously over 1 h or placebo. Patients were treated within 12 h of the onset of symptoms. Overall mortality at 21 days was 13% in the control group and 10.7% in the treated group (relative risk 0.81, 95% CI 0.72–0.90, $p = 0.0002$). The greatest relative risk reduction was in those patients treated within 3 h of the onset of symptoms. At 1 year, mortality was 17.2% in the streptokinase group and 19% in the control group (relative risk 0.90, 95% C 0.84–0.97, $p = 0.008$). The reduction in mortality was only seen in those patients treated within 6 h of the onset of symptoms.

The beneficial effects of thrombolysis seen in GISSI-I were confirmed with the publication of ISIS-2,[6] which involved the randomization of 17 178 patients to receive aspirin, streptokinase, both or neither. The 5-week vascular mortality among the streptokinase- and placebo-treated patients was 9.2% and

12.0% respectively (odds reduction 25%, 95% CI 18–32%, $p < 0.00001$). Further, the addition of aspirin was found to be synergistic, with a 5-week mortality of 8.0%, compared to 13.2% among patients treated with neither agent (odds reduction 42.0%, 95% CI 34.0–50.0%).

The results of GISSI-I and ISIS-2, taken with those of ISAM (using streptokinase),[39] AIMS (using APSAC)[49] and ASSET (using tPA),[50] form a robust collection of evidence supporting the routine use of thrombolysis in the setting of acute myocardial infarction.

The Fibrinolytic Therapy Trialists' (FTT) Collaborative Group has performed a comprehensive review of the nine largest randomized trials, each enrolling more than 1000 patients. Taken together, they combine the data on over 58 000 patients randomized to receive thrombolysis or placebo. Overall, the results indicate an 18% reduction in short-term mortality. However, this is increased to 25% if the 45% of patients presenting with ST segment elevation or LBBB on an ECG are considered as a subset. What is also apparent is the time-dependent factor following the onset of symptoms. The number of lives saved per 1000 patients treated was 35 in those treated within the first hour, 25 between 2 and 3 h, 19 between 4 and 6 h, and 16 between 7 and 12 h. Whether the administration of thrombolysis beyond

6 h was worthwhile remained controversial, and two trials specifically addressed this issue.

EMERAS (Estudio Multicentrico Estreptoquinasa Republicus de America der Sur)[51] studied the use of streptokinase. In the trial, 4534 patients presenting with acute myocardial infarction at >6 h and <24 h were randomized to receive 1.5 million units of streptokinase or placebo infused over 1 h. There was no difference in the in-hospital mortality (11.9% with streptokinase versus 12.4% with placebo). There was a trend towards reduced mortality in patients presenting between 7 and 12 h after the onset of symptoms (11.7% versus 13.2%). One-year mortality was similar between the streptokinase and placebo groups.

In the LATE Study,[52] 5711 patients aged greater than 18 years presenting between 6 and 24 h after the onset of a myocardial infarction were randomized to receive intravenous alteplase (r-tPA) 10-mg bolus or matching placebo. Thirty-five-day mortality for patients treated 6–12 h after the onset of symptoms was 8.9% versus 12.0% in the alteplase and placebo groups respectively (95% CI 6.3–45%, $p = 0.02$). There was no significant difference in mortality in patients treated at >12 h after the onset of symptoms.

It has been suggested that patients presenting

up to 12 h after the onset of symptoms of myocardial infarction benefit from thrombolysis, and treatment should be offered until this time unless there are contraindications to treatment. Routine administration of thrombolysis beyond 12 h is not supported by clinical evidence. However, each case should be considered on merit, and the persistence of ischaemic cardiac pain with ECG evidence supporting the use of thrombolysis would justify the use of such therapy even in patients whose initial symptoms appeared more than 12 h before assessment.

In order to accelerate the process of restoration of coronary perfusion, pre-hospital thrombolysis has been considered. Two studies have looked at this issue. The first, a small study carried out in the Grampian region of Scotland,[53] randomized 311 patients to home thrombolysis or thrombolysis after arrival in hospital. Home treatment led to a thrombolytic agent being given earlier by a median of 130 min. After 3 months, the mortality in those treated at home was 8% compared with 15.5% for those treated in hospital.

However, a much larger study, EMIP (European Myocardial Infarction Project),[54] randomized 5569 patients to receive anistreplase either at home or after hospitalization. The 30-day mortality rates were 9.7% (anistreplase at home) and 11.1% (anistreplase in hospital), a difference which was not statistically significant. Therefore, although both of the studies demonstrated the safety of pre-hospital thrombolysis, the evidence supporting its routine use is not compelling. It may have a role, depending on local factors, such as the potential delay before hospitalization in rural areas.

Once the mortality benefit of thrombolysis was established, the era of placebo-controlled trials came to an end. It was no longer ethically acceptable to withhold this life-saving therapy. Attention then switched to determining which thrombolytic agent would provide the most benefit.

Four thrombolytic agents have been assessed. Urokinase, a naturally occurring plasminogen activator isolated from human urine and human embryonic kidney cells, has been used as a thrombolytic for over three decades. Although potentially less antigenic than streptokinase, its high cost and apparent lack of superior efficacy over streptokinase has meant that its use has been limited to intracoronary thrombolysis. Streptokinase is a non-enzymatic protein produced by β-haemolytic streptococci. It activates plasminogen indirectly by a three-step process. Most individuals have measurable neutralizing antibodies, presumably acquired as a result of previous streptococcal infection. These antibodies are overcome by giving sufficient streptokinase to overcome their neutralizing effect. However, following streptokinase administration, their titre rapidly rises and remains elevated for up to 4 years. Renewed usage is, therefore, no longer recommended. Anisoylated plasminogen–streptokinase complex (APSAC) is synthetically constructed and, because of its longer half-life (70 min), allows bolus injection. This agent was used in the pre-hospital trials of thrombolysis. Tissue plasminogen activator is a naturally occurring plasminogen activator, initially isolated from the human melanoma cell line, but which for commercial use is produced by recombinant DNA technology.

Early angiographic studies suggested that tPA was more efficacious than other agents in terms of infarct-related artery patency. This was investigated in three large outcome studies which compared commonly used thrombolytic agents.

The first, GISSI 2,[26] compared intravenous streptokinase (1.5 MU/h) with tPA (50 mg/h + 40 mg/2 h). Over 20 000 patients were randomized. All patients received aspirin, and half in each group were randomized to receive subcutaneous heparin. Results showed no difference in in-hospital mortality, which was 8.9% for tPA and 8.5% for streptokinase. More strokes occurred with tPA (1.3%) than with streptokinase (0.9%).

ISIS 3[27] was a three-armed trial comparing streptokinase (1.5 MU/h), tPA (0.04 MU/kg bolus, 0.36 MU/kg/per hour, 0.067 MU/kg/per hour for 3 h), and APSAC (30 U/3 min); 41 299 patients with suspected myocardial infarction were randomized. Again, each patient received aspirin, and half in each group were randomized to receive subcutaneous heparin. No significant difference was found between thrombolytic agents in terms of reinfarction or 30-day mortality. tPA was associated with fewer allergic reactions than streptokinase but with a higher rate of non-cerebral haemorrhage. Stroke occurred in 1.04% of the streptokinase group, compared with 1.39% of the tPA group.

Therefore, a meta-analysis of GISSI 2 and ISIS 3 combining over 48 000 patients suggests no difference in efficacy between the routinely used thrombolytic agents.

However, both of these studies were criticized in that neither used tPA in its accelerated form and given in combination with intravenous heparin. Certainly, in terms of angiographic data, this seemed to be the most efficacious mode of giving tPA. To address this issue, the GUSTO I trial was performed. Patients in this trial were randomized to receive one of four therapeutic interventions: (1) streptokinase 1.5 MU/h + intravenous heparin; (2) 'accelerated' tPA + intravenous heparin; (3) combination streptokinase 1.0 MU/h + intravenous tPA 1 mg/kg per hour; (4) streptokinase 1.5 MU + subcutaneous heparin. All patients received aspirin and a beta-blocker unless contraindicated.

Thirty-day mortality was 7.2% for the streptokinase + subcutaneous heparin group, 7.4% for the streptokinase + intravenous heparin group, 6.3% for 'accelerated' tPA + intravenous heparin, and 7.0% for the combination group. Thus, there was a 14% reduction in 30-day mortality for accelerated tPA compared to the other streptokinase-treated groups (95% CI 5.9–21.3%). Haemorrhagic stroke occurred in 0.49%, 0.54%, 0.72% and 0.94% in the four groups respectively ($p = 0.03$ for the difference between tPA and streptokinase). It therefore appears that tPA given in its accelerated form with intravenous heparin does offer an advantage when compared with intravenous streptokinase. However, this is at a higher cost of intracranial haemorrhage.

It is difficult, therefore, to give clear recommendations on the choice of thrombolytic agent, especially given that local financial factors play a part in the choice of agent used. Those at highest risk would seem to benefit most from the added benefit of tPA over streptokinase. However, the risk of intracranial haemorrhage increases with age

>65 years, body weight <70 kg, systemic hypertension (systolic BP > 180 mmHg) and tPA as opposed to streptokinase.

Perhaps it should be emphasized that it is the administration of thrombolysis as rapidly as possible which is able to determine a patient's outcome, way and above which actual thrombolytic agent is chosen. The GUSTO I investigators developed a regression model to illustrate the relative importance of clinical characteristics for 30-day mortality in thrombolytic-treated patients. The 'mortality pyramid' (Fig. 7.3) demonstrates that much greater proportions of the risks of mortality are contributed by blood pressure and heart rate at presentation than precisely which thrombolytic agent was used (for example, the use of tPA contributed less than 1% to the proportional effect on mortality after adjusting for other clinical variables).

The benefits of thrombolysis are, therefore, well established; however, there are two major drawbacks to its use. First thrombolysis may result in unwanted haemorrhage and, in particular, intracranial bleeding. Second, the early and sustained patency of infarct-related arteries is less than optimal with current regimens in common clinical use. Angiographic data have established that, even in its most potent currently utilized form, thrombolysis achieves only 75–85% infarct-related artery patency. Currently, there are

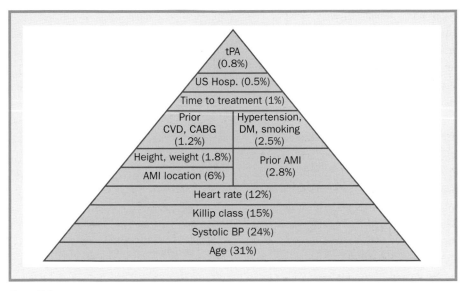

Figure 7.3
Influence of clinical characteristics on 30-day mortality after acute myocardial infarction (AMI) in patients treated with thrombolytic agents based on experience from the GUSTO trial. CABG, coronary artery bypass graft; CVD, cardiovascular disease; DM, diabetes mellitus.

two approaches aimed at addressing these issues.

Molecular modification and protein conjugation of tPA has produced fibrinolytics which have (1) increased fibrin specificity, and (2) altered pharmacokinetics.[55] This enables these agents to be given as a bolus injection in order to achieve more rapid infarct-related artery patency[56] and, with increased clot specificity, a reduction in unwanted haemorrhage. These agents are also modified in order to increase resistance to plasminogen activator inhibitor-1 and so reduce their clearance from the circulation.

The second approach to maintaining artery patency and reducing unwanted effects is the use of adjunctive therapy. The use of antiplatelet agents and direct thrombin inhibitors as adjuncts to thrombolysis is being investigated.[57] One approach has been the use of these agents to achieve similar rates of infarct-related artery patency but with lower doses of thrombolytic agents, with the intention of reducing unwanted bleeding events.

The development of new thrombolytic agents and the use of adjunctive therapy has again led to a new era of thrombolytic trials. The benefits potentially offered by each new approach are likely to be small, and huge numbers of patients are required in order to demonstrate improved clinical outcome. This has led to a new approach in the assessment of new thrombolytic regimens. So-called 'equivalence trials' involve the comparison of a new agent or regimen with a currently accepted therapeutic approach in order to show statistical 'equivalence' in terms of clinical outcome. If the new agent or approach has the added benefit of fewer unwanted effects or perhaps reduced cost, it has a demonstrated advantage over the therapy with which it is being compared. INJECT[58] is such a trial, and compared streptokinase with a modified tPA, r-PA; 6010 patients were randomized to receive either r-PA or streptokinase. Patients were followed up for 6 months. Thirty-five-day and 6-month mortality were similar in the both groups but hypotension and allergic reactions were more common in the streptokinase-treated group.

Similar trials investigating other tPA mutants and various adjunctive therapies are currently underway and will no doubt modify the way in which we use this life-saving therapy. Enhancement of this therapeutic intervention provides a path to the future. While primary coronary angioplasty offers much to selected individuals where it is available, thrombolysis with or without adjunctive therapy is going to remain the life-saving intervention which is available to the vast majority of patients presenting with acute myocardial infarction.

References

1. Davies MJ, Thomas AC, Plaque fissuring—the course of acute myocardial infarction, sudden ischaemic death and crescendo angina, *Br Heart J* 1985; **53**: 363.

2. Falk E, Coronary thrombosis: pathogenesis and clinical manifestations, *Am J Cardiol* 1991; **68**: 28B.

3. Willerson JT, Conversion from acute coronary heart disease syndromes: the role of platelets and platelet products, *Tex Heart Inst J* 1995; **22**: 13.

4. Falk E, Shah PK, Fuster V, Coronary plaque disruption, *Circulation* 1995; **92**: 657.

5. Kragel AH, Reddy SG, Wittes JT et al, Morphometric analysis of the composition of atherosclerotic plaques in the four major epicardial coronary arteries in acute myocardial infarction and in sudden coronary death, *Circulation* 1989; **80**: 1747.

6. ISIS 2 (Second International Study of Infarct Survival) Collaborative Group, Randomised trial of intravenous streptokinase, oral aspirin, both or neither among 17,187 cases of suspected acute myocardial infarction, *Lancet* 1988; **2**: 349–60.

7. Antiplatelets Trialists Collaboration, Collaborative overview of randomised trials of antiplatelet therapy. Prevention of death, myocardial infarction and stroke by prolonged antiplatelet therapy in various categories of patients, *Br Med J* 1994; **308**: 81–106.

8. Patrono C, Aspirin as an antiplatelet drug, *N Engl J Med* 1994; **330**: 1287–94.

9. Szczeklik A, Krzanowski M, Gora P, Randwan J, Antiplatelet drugs and generation of thrombin in clotting blood, *Blood* 1992; **80**: 2006.

10. Szczeklik A, Thrombin generation in myocardial infarction and hypercholesterolaemia; effects of aspirin, *Thromb Haemost* 1995; **74**: 77.

11. Meade EA, Smith WL, Dewitt DL, Differential inhibition of prostaglandin endoperoxide anti-inflammatory drugs, *J Biol Chem* 1993; **268**: 610.

12. Patrignani P, Filabozzi P, Patrono C, Selective cumulative inhibition of platelet thromboxane production by low dose aspirin in healthy subjects, *J Clin Invest* 1982; **69**: 1366–72.

13. Reilly IAG, Fitzgerald GA, Inhibition of thromboxane formation in-vivo and ex-vivo: implications for therapy with platelet inhibitory drugs, *Blood* 1987; **69**: 180–6.

14. Berglund U, Wallentin L, Persistent inhibition of platelet function during longterm treatment with 75 mg acetylsalicylic acid daily in men with unstable coronary artery disease, *Eur Heart J* 1991; **12**: 428–33.

15. Link KP, The discovery of dicumarol and its sequels, *Circulation* 1959; **19**: 97–107.

16. Chalmers TC, Matta RJ, Smith H et al, Evidence favouring the use of anticoagulants in the hospital phase of acute myocardial infarction, *New Engl J Med* 1977; **297**: 1091–6.

17. MacMahon S, Collins R, Knight C et al, Reduction in major morbidity and mortality by heparin in acute myocardial infarction, *Circulation* 1988; **78**(suppl II): 98.

18. Vaitkus PT, Berlin JA, Schwartz JS et al, Stroke complicating acute myocardial infarction: a meta-analysis of risk modification by anticoagulant and thrombolytic therapy, *Arch Intern Med* 1992; **152**: 2020.

19. Fitzgerald DJ, Catella F, Roy L et al, Marked platelet activation in vivo after intravenous streptokinase in patients with acute myocardial infarction, *Circulation* 1988; **77**: 142–50.

20. Eisenberg PR, Sobel BE, Jaffe AS, Activation of prothrombin accompanying thrombolysis with recombinant tissue-type plasminogen activator, *JACC* 1992; **19**: 1065–9.

21. Owen JM, Friedman KD, Grossman BA et al, Thrombolytic therapy with tissue type plasminogen activator or streptokinase induced transient thrombin activity, *Blood* 1988; **72**: 616–20.

22. Genser N, Mair J, Maier J et al, Thrombin generation during infusion of tissue-plasminogen activator, *Lancet* 1993; **341**: 1038.

23. Garabedian HD, Gold HK, Coronary thrombolysis, conjunctive heparin infusion and the effect on systemic thrombin activity, *Circulation* 1992; **85**: 1205–7.

24. Anderson HV, Willeson JT, Thrombolysis in acute myocardial infarction, *N Engl J Med* 1993; **329**: 703–9.

25. The SCATI Group, Randomised control trial of subcutaneous calcium-heparin in acute myocardial infarction, *Lancet* 1989; **2**: 182–9.

26. Gruppo Italiano per lo Studio della Sopravvivenza Neu Infarcto Miocardico,

GISSI-2, a factorial randomised trial of alteplase versus streptokinase and heparin versus no heparin among 12,490 patients with acute myocardial infarction, *Lancet* 1990; **1336**: 65–71.

27. ISIS-3 (Third International Study of Infarct Survival) Collaborative Study Group, ISIS-3: a randomised comparison of streptokinase versus tissue plasminogen activator versus anistreplase and of aspirin plus heparin versus aspirin alone among 41,299 cases of suspected acute myocardial infarction, *Lancet* 1992; **339**: 753–70.

28. The GUSTO Investigators, An international randomised trial comparing four thrombolytic strategies for acute myocardial infarction, *N Engl J Med* 1993; **329**: 673.

29. LATE (Late Assessment of Thrombolytic Efficacy) Study Group, Late Assessment of thrombolytic therapy (LATE) Study with alteplase 6–24 hours after the onset of myocardial infarction, *Lancet* 1993; **342**: 759.

30. Bleich SD, Nichols TC, Schumacher RR et al, Effect of heparin on coronary arterial patency after thrombolysis with tissue plasminogen activator in acute myocardial infarction, *Am J Cardiol* 1990; **66**: 1412–17.

31. Hsia J, Hamilton WP, Kleiman N et al, A comparison between heparin and low-dose aspirin as adjunctive therapy with tissue plasminogen activator for acute myocardial infarction, *N Engl J Med* 1990; **323**: 1433–7.

32. De Bono DP, Simoons MI, Tijssen J et al, Effect of early intravenous heparin on coronary patency, infarct size and bleeding complications after alteplase thrombolysis: results of a randomised double blind European Co-operative Study Group trial, *Br Heart J* 1992; **67**: 122.

33. Theroux P, Waters D, Lam J et al, Reactivation of unstable angina after the discontinuation of heparin, *N Engl J Med* 1992; **327**: 141.

34. Hassan WM, Flaker GC, Feutz C et al, Improved anticoagulation with a weight adjusted heparin normogram in patients with acute coronary syndromes: a randomised trial, *J Throm Thrombol* 1996; **2**: 245.

35. Vaitkus P, Barnathan E, Embolic potential, prevention and management of mural thrombus complicating anterior myocardial infarction: a meta-analysis, *J Am Coll Cardiol* 1993; **22**: 1004.

36. Meeting Highlights: AHA 68th Scientific Sessions, TIMI 9B: Heparin versus hirudin as adjunctive therapy for thrombolysis in acute myocardial infarction, *Circulation* 1996; **93**: 843.

37. Canon CP, McCabe CH, Henry TD et al, A pilot trial of recombinant desulfafohirudin compared with heparin in conjunction with tPA and aspirin for acute myocardial infarction: results of the thrombolysis and myocardial infarction (TIMI 5) trial, *J Am Coll Cardiol* 1994; **23**: 993–1003.

38. Gruppo Italiano Pr Lo Studio Della Streptokinasi Neu'infarct, Miocardico (GISSI): effectiveness of intravenous thrombolytic treatment in acute myocardial infarction, *Lancet* 1986; **1**: 397.

39. ISAM-2 (Intravenous Streptokinase in Acute Myocardial Infarction) Study Group, A prospective trial of intravenous streptokinase in acute myocardial infarction, *N Engl J Med* 1986; **314**: 1465.

40. Fibrinolytic Therapy Trialists (FTT) Collaborative Group Indications for fibrinolytic therapy in suspected acute myocardial infarction: collaborative overview

of early mortality and major morbidity results from all randomised trials of more than 1,000 patients, *Lancet* 1994; **343**: 311.

41. Reimer KA, Lowe JA, Rasmusen NM et al, The wavefront phenomenon of ischaemic cell death: myocardial infarct size versus duration of coronary occlusion in dogs, *Circulation* 1977; **56**: 786–94.

42. Reimer KA, Jennings RB, The 'wavefront' phenomenon of myocardial ischaemic cell death, *Lab Invest* 1979; **40**: 633–44.

43. Rentrop P, Smith H, Painter L et al, Changes in left ventricular ejection fraction after intracoronary thrombolytic therapy: results of the Registry of the European Society of Cardiology, *Circulation* 1983; **68**(suppl I):155–160.

44. Gibbons RJ, Christian TJ, Hopfenspirger M et al, Myocardium at risk and infarct size after thrombolysis therapy for acute myocardial infarction: implications for the design of randomised trials of acute intervention, *J Am Coll Cardiol* 1994; **24**: 616–23.

45. Cherbero JH, Knattenid G, Roberts R et al, Thrombolysis in Myocardial Infarction (TIMI) Trial; Phase I: a comparison between intravenous tissue plasminogen activator and intravenous streptokinase. Clinical findings through hospital discharge, *Circulation* 1987; **76**: 142–54.

46. The GUSTO Angiographic Investigators, The comparative effects of tissue plasminogen activator, streptokinase or both on coronary artery patency, ventricular function and survival after myocardial infarction, *N Engl J Med* 1993; **329**: 1615.

47. Lenderink T, Simoons ML, van Es GA et al, Benefits of thrombolytic therapy is sustained throughout five years and is related to TIMI perfusion grade 3 but not grade 2 flow at discharge, *Circulation* 1995; **92**: 1110.

48. Fletcher AP, Alkjaersig N, Smymiotis FE et al, The treatment of patients suffering with early myocardial infarction with massive and prolonged streptokinase therapy, *Trans Assoc Am Physicians* 1958; **71**: 287.

49. AIMS Trial Study Group, Effect of intravenous APSAC on the mortality after acute myocardial infarction: preliminary report of a placebo-controlled clinical trial, *Lancet* 1988; **1**: 545.

50. Wilcox RG, von der Lippe G, Olsson CG et al, Trial of tissue plasminogen activator for mortality reduction in acute myocardial infarction: Anglo-Scandinavian Study of Early Thrombolysis (ASSET), *Lancet* 1988; **1**: 525.

51. EMERAS Collaborative Group, Randomised trial of late thrombolysis in patients with suspected myocardial infarction, *Lancet* 1993; **343**: 767–72.

52. LATE (Late Assessment of Thrombolytic Efficacy) Study Group, Late assessment of thrombolytic therapy study alteplase 6–24 hours after the onset of myocardial infarction, *Lancet* 1993; **342**: 759.

53. GREAT Group, Feasibility, safety and efficacy of domicillary thrombolysis by general practitioners, *Br Med J* 1992; **305**: 548–53.

54. The European Myocardial Infarction Project Group, Prehospital thrombolytic therapy in patients with suspected myocardial infarction, *N Engl J Med* 1993; **329**: 383–9.

55. Vaughan D, Loscatzo J, New directions in thrombolytic therapy: molecular mutants and biochemical conjugates, *Trends Cardiovasc Med* 1991; **1**: 36.

56. TIMI 10, TNK—Tissue plasminogen activator in acute myocardial infarction. TIMI 10A dose-ranging trial, *Circulation* 1997; **95**: 351–6.

57. The Argatroban in Myocardial Infarction Study (AMI), To assess the effect of adding argatroban, a direct thrombin inhibitor, to streptokinase thrombolysis in patients with acute myocardial infarction, *J Am Coll Cardiol* 1997; **30**: 1–7.

58. Randomised, double blind comparison of reteplase double bolus administration with streptokinase in acute myocardial infarction (INJECT): trial to investigate equivalence, *Lancet* 1995; **346**: 329–36.

Other medical treatment

Peter F Ludman

8

Beta-blockers

There have been many proposed mechanisms for the benefits of beta-blockade in the acute and chronic treatment of myocardial infarction. Beta-blocker therapy results in a reduction in myocardial oxygen demand (reducing heart rate, blood pressure and contractility). There may be protection from the arrhythmogenic and hypokalaemic effects of catecholamines, inhibition of platelet aggregation, an improvement in subendocardial perfusion (partly due to prolongation of diastole) and a shift from glucose to free fatty acid metabolism, enabling more ATP production.[1] Evidence that these theoretical benefits actually occur in humans is patchy.

Before the widespread use of thrombolysis, it was shown that long-term treatment with timolol[2] and propranolol[3] following acute myocardial infarction reduced mortality. In these studies, treatment was started after 1–3 weeks of acute myocardial infarction, and at follow-up of about 2–3 years there was a mortality reduction from 13.9% to 7.7% with timolol and from 10% to 7% with propranolol. Intravenous beta-blockers also appeared to provide survival benefit when given early to patients presenting with acute myocardial infarction (Table 8.1). The Goteborg metoprolol study[4] showed a 36% reduction in mortality (from 8.9% to 5.7%) at 3 months. Patients were treated with intravenous metoprolol within 12 h of chest pain onset. Two much larger trials supported this finding. The MIAMI trial[5] showed a trend to reduction in 15-day mortality of 13% (4.9–4.3%, p = NS) with metoprolol, and a 15% mortality reduction was achieved with intravenous atenolol in ISIS-1[6] (4.6–3.9%, p < 0.04). Nevertheless, because of anxieties

Table 8.1
Summary of the major trials of beta-blocker therapy for acute myocardial infarction.

Trial	N	Drug and timing	Main outcomes (treatment versus control)
No thrombolysis			
Goteberg metoprolol group[4]	1395	Metoprolol 15 mg IV over 6 min 50 mg PO after 15 min, 6-hourly for 48 h 100 mg PO bd for 90 days	Total mortality at 90/7 5.7% versus 8.9% (p < 0.03)
MIAMI[5]	5778	Metoprolol 15 mg IV over 6 min, then 100 mg bd PO	Mortality at 15 days 4.3% versus 4.9% (p = 0.29)
ISIS-1[6]	16027	Atenolol 5–10 mg IV, then 100 mg od PO for 7 days	Vascular mortality (a) at 7 days 3.9% versus 4.6% (p < 0.04) (b) at 1 year 10.7% versus 12% (p < 0.01)
Post thrombolysis			
TIMI-II B[12]	1434	Metoprolol 15 mg IV over 6 min 50 mg PO after 15 min, 12-hourly for 12 h 100 mg PO bd to continue	Global EF at 6 days 51.0% versus 50.1% (p = 0.22) Mortality at 6 days 2.4% versus 2.4% (p = 0.98)

EF, ejection fraction.

about adverse effects, both these trials only recruited patients with a good prognosis (note the ≈5% mortality in the placebo arms), making the absolute benefits small. A recent retrospective analysis of the Goteborg study suggests that those patients with mild to moderate heart failure before randomization may gain most benefit (with a mortality of 10% versus 19% at 3 months).[7]

When the mechanism of benefit was studied in ISIS-1,[8] it was found that the survival curves separated at 24 h, and thereafter remained parallel. The benefit appeared to be due to a reduction in the incidence of myocardial rupture. This concept was given indirect support when looking at the results of the MIAMI trial, which also showed little evidence of further benefit after early divergence of the survival curves. If benefit were due to limitation in infarct size (the other possible explanation of benefit), then a late reduction in mortality might have been expected, as has since been observed in the thrombolytic trials. The importance of trying to reduce rupture rates was highlighted by a large autopsy study looking at rates over a 16-year period.[9] Data in this large number of patients (intravenous beta-blockade was not used at any time) show that the rate of myocardial rupture in patients admitted with myocardial infarction remained unchanged at about 4% from 1977 to 1992. As overall hospital mortality

declines towards 10%, rupture assumes greater relative importance.

With the advent of reperfusion therapy, the value of acute beta-blockade was unclear. Though the overall rate of myocardial rupture does not appear to have changed, it seems to occur earlier in the evolution of infarction when thrombolytic agents are used.[10] Perhaps beta-blockade would be particularly beneficial in patients treated with thrombolytics. In addition, animal work had demonstrated that immediate beta-blockade could augment myocardial salvage by thrombolysis.[11]

The TIMI II-B study assessed treatment with tissue plasminogen activator (tPA) and intravenous metoprolol.[12] The results were disappointing. There was no benefit in left ventricular function and no reduction in mortality when comparing those treated with immediate rather than deferred (6–8 days) metoprolol. Furthermore, there was no reduction in the incidence of myocardial rupture. There was a reduction in the incidence of recurrent chest pain (18.8% versus 24.1%, $p < 0.02$) and reinfarction (2.7% versus 5.1%, $p = 0.02$), but this difference was not maintained at 1-year follow-up. More recent evidence comes from a small study using carvedilol (a non-selective beta-blocker with additional vasodilating properties caused by alpha$_1$-blockade) in acute myocardial infarction, suggesting benefit.[13]

Some of the different outcomes of these trials may relate to differences in the characteristics of the beta-blocker used. The hypothesis that degree of lipid solubility of these drugs may be important is given some support when looking at combined information derived from both the primary and secondary prevention trials. Those drugs that have been shown to improve longer-term outlook are lipophilic agents (e.g. timolol, propranolol and metoprolol). These can cross the blood–brain barrier and cause central vagal stimulation. There is substantial evidence both in animals and humans that high vagal tone is associated with improved outcome, particularly in chronic heart failure. In contrast, hydrophilic agents (e.g. atenolol and sotalol) have been less beneficial. While acute rupture may have been reduced by atenolol in ISIS-1, evidence for longer-term benefit from this drug (albeit from primary prevention trials) is lacking;[14] indeed, this may explain the lack of continued divergence of the survival curves in ISIS-1 after the first 24 h. The UK sotalol study[15] is the only large study of a beta-blocker that has not shown an effect on sudden death more marked than an effect on overall mortality. Sotalol's effect as a class III anti-arrhythmic agent may be another explanation for this finding.

There have been concerns about potential adverse effects when intravenous beta-blockade is combined with thrombolysis in the setting of acute myocardial infarction. Data are now available from several large studies of thrombolysis where intravenous beta-blockade was used as part of routine therapy. An example is GISSI-2,[16] where intravenous atenolol was given as standard therapy. While acknowledging that this was not a randomized treatment strategy, the data were encouraging. About 45% of patients were deemed clinically suitable for acute beta-blocker treatment.[17] Those receiving beta-blocker had a lower incidence of advanced atrioventricular block (4.3% versus 12.3%), less sustained ventricular tachycardia (2.8% versus 4.5%), ventricular fibrillation (4.9% versus 12%) and heart failure (7.1% versus 8%). There was an increase in transient hypotension in those treated with streptokinase versus tPA, but there was no difference in sustained hypotension (4.6%).

In conclusion, there is good evidence to support the use of immediate intravenous beta-blockers in patients who do not receive reperfusion therapy. Though the largest trials only enrolled low-risk patients, higher-risk patients may have more to gain. There may be some benefit in patients who do receive thrombolysis, but this has not yet been convincingly demonstrated. In patients without contraindications to intravenous beta-blockade, this treatment does not appear to be associated with significant hazard. Thus in the current treatment of acute myocardial infarction it seems reasonable to recommend early (but not necessarily immediate) treatment with a lipophilic beta-blocker. Given the increasingly robust evidence regarding beta-blocker benefit in chronic heart failure, and acknowledged progression from acute infarction to chronic impaired left ventricular function, beta-blocker treatment should be considered in all infarct survivors. Those with large infarcts and impaired left ventricular function probably have the most to gain.

Calcium antagonists

Short-acting nifedipine

In the treatment of acute myocardial infarction it is quite clear that short-acting nifedipine does not confer significant therapeutic benefit (and it may be deleterious). This lack of benefit is found in all patients, male or female, Q-wave or non-Q-wave infarction, in the presence or absence of concomitant thrombolytic agents or beta-blockers and irrespective of overall risk.

There are many trials supporting these conclusions, of which a few will be discussed. The trial of early nifedipine in acute myocardial infarction (TRENT)[18] enrolled 4491 patients with suspected myocardial infarction. About 64% actually sustained infarction. In this group, mortality at 1 month was 9.3% (placebo) versus 10.2% (nifedipine), which was not statistically significant. In the Norwegian Nifedipine Multicentre Trial of 227 patients treated at 5.5 h (mean) of infarction, there was no significant difference in infarct size as determined by enzyme rise,[19] but there was a trend to increased mortality. In the Secondary Prevention Reinfarction Israeli Nifedipine Trial II (SPRINT-II),[20] 1006 patients judged to be having high-risk myocardial infarctions were treated, usually within 3 h of admission. Mortality was 18.7% among those randomized to nifedipine and 15.6% in the patients randomized to placebo. This reflected an increased mortality of 7.8% as compared with 5.5% during the first 6 days in the nifedipine and placebo groups, respectively (p = NS). In a smaller trial by Muller et al,[21] treatment was started within a mean of 4.6 h in 105 patients with threatened and 66 with acute myocardial infarction. The incidence of progression to infarction among patients with threatened myocardial infarction was not significantly altered by nifedipine (36 of 48 (75%) for placebo-treated and 43 of 57 (75%) for nifedipine-treated patients). Among the 171 eligible patients randomly assigned to drug or placebo, 6-month mortality did not differ significantly (8.5% for placebo versus 10.1% for nifedipine, p = NS), but mortality in the 2 weeks after randomization was significantly higher for nifedipine-treated patients.

There are currently no data to clarify the role of the slow-release preparations of nifedipine, or the other dihydropyridines (such as felodipine or amlodipine).

Heart rate-slowing calcium channel blockers

Investigations into the role of diltiazem and verapamil in the treatment of acute myocardial infarction have been more encouraging. The larger trials include the Danish Verapamil Infarction Trials (DAVIT) I[22] and II,[23] the Multicentre Diltiazem Postinfarction Trial (MDPIT)[24] and the Diltiazem Reinfarction Study.[25] It is of note that these trials were all conducted before the widespread use of either aspirin or thrombolysis.

The Diltiazem Reinfarction Study assessed 576 patients with non-Q-wave myocardial infarction; treatment started at 24–72 h from the onset of symptoms. There was a reduction in early reinfarction and in refractory angina, but no change in mortality at 14 days. There was a 61% use of concomitant beta-blockade. The MDPIT study was much larger, enrolling 2466 patients, treated 3–15 days after infarction. Though there was no overall difference in mortality, the neutral effect reflected a diltiazem-related reduction in cardiac events in patients without left ventricular dysfunction, and an increase in events in those with left ventricular function.

Twenty per cent of this study population had pulmonary congestion, and in this subgroup the hazard ratio for a cardiac event was 1.41. In the 80% of patients without evidence of congestion, the hazard ratio was 0.77.

The DAVIT I study was designed to assess the effect of verapamil given very early in the course of myocardial infarction. There was no difference between treatment and placebo in mortality or reinfarction rates at 6 months. Nevertheless, retrospective analysis suggested that benefit might occur between days 22 and 180. This was the major stimulus to the DAVIT II study, where verapamil was started later, in the second week after admission, and continued for 18 months; 1775 patients were randomized, and there was a small reduction in mortality (11.1% versus 13.8%, $p = 0.11$) and a larger reduction in major event rates (18.0% versus 21.6%, $p = 0.03$) at 18 months. In patients with heart failure, there was no significant deleterious or beneficial effect (mortality 17.9% versus 17.5%), but in those without heart failure, there was a significant reduction in mortality (7.7% versus 11.8%, $p = 0.02$) and major events (14.6% versus 19.7%, $p = 0.01$).

In both DAVIT II and MDPIT, subgroup analyses suggested that those patients without heart failure, but with hypertension, derived the most benefit from treatment with verapamil and diltiazem respectively.

The research above was conducted before the widespread use of aspirin or reperfusion therapy, and with immediate-release preparations of medication. Given those caveats, the data would support the use of verapamil and diltiazem started a few days after myocardial infarction, in patients with no evidence of cardiac failure, in whom beta-blockers are contraindicated. It may be that those with hypertension gain the most benefit.

INTERCEPT, the Incomplete Infarction Trial of European Research Collaborators Evaluating Prognosis Post Thrombolysis (diltiazem),[26] is due to publish in 1998–99. This will be the first large prospective study to assess the value of sustained-release diltiazem in patients receiving thrombolytic therapy for first myocardial infarction. The 6-month cumulative occurrence of cardiac death, recurrent non-fatal acute myocardial infarction and refractory angina will be measured. This trial will hopefully answer some of the outstanding questions about the role of 'modern' calcium channel blockers in acute myocardial infarction.

Nitrates

The endothelium of vessels is now recognized as playing a central role in modulating smooth muscle function and growth. Endothelium-derived relaxing factor (EDRF) has been identified as nitric oxide (NO) or a closely related compound. Nitric oxide is a potent vasorelaxant (via guanylate cyclase) and is formed in endothelium from the guanidine nitrogen terminus of L-arginine by the enzyme NO synthase. There are several drugs that increase NO levels near the plasma membrane of smooth muscle cells and so cause vessel dilatation, mimicking the effects of endogenous EDRF. While sodium nitroprusside releases NO spontaneously, there are also three organic nitrates in use. Isosorbide dinitrate (ISDN) is extensively metabolized in the liver to form two active metabolites, isosorbide-2 and isosorbide-5 mononitrate. Isosorbide-5 mononitrate (ISMN) preparations do not undergo hepatic metabolic change and are therefore fully bioavailable. Glyceryl trinitrate (GTN) is rapidly metabolized to inactive metabolites and has a very short half-life.

There are many theoretical benefits of nitrate therapy in acute myocardial infarction. Nitrates reduce myocardial work by venodilatation and hence reduction of preload and also of peripheral vascular resistance and blood pressure. Nitrates also cause epicardial coronary artery dilatation. While some coronary stenoses are rigid, many remain responsive to vasoactive stimuli. If coronary spasm is associated with an acute coronary syndrome, nitrates can cause dilatation and so improve anterograde coronary perfusion. Dilatation of coronary collateral vessels has also been demonstrated, and NO also inhibits platelet aggregation and adhesion to endothelium. Early work in both animals and humans showed a reduction in infarct size, improvement in left ventricular function and improvement in ventricular remodelling.[27] A meta-analysis of a number of small clinical trials suggested the possibility of mortality reduction of the order of 35%,[28] but there were wide confidence limits.

Two large trials, however, have failed to confirm the hoped-for benefits. In GISSI-3,[29] 19 394 patients were randomized to assess the potential benefits of lisinopril, organic nitrate or a combination, in a randomized factorial design. Intravenous GTN was given from time of presentation for 24 h, followed by transdermal GTN for the next 6 weeks. There were no significant differences at 6 weeks in mortality, rates of reinfarction or revascularization procedures. There was an unexpected small but significant excess of stroke. Nevertheless, the safety of widespread but empirical GTN use in the acute phase of myocardial infarction was confirmed. In the ISIS-4 trial,[30] almost 60 000 patients were randomized to 1 month of treatment with oral controlled-release ISMN. This was started within a few hours of thrombolysis treatment. The results showed no significant mortality benefit at the 5-week end-point, and no particular subgroup appeared to derive benefit. Again, the results supported the safety of nitrate use.

In conclusion, in spite of many compelling arguments about the theoretical benefits of nitrate therapy, there is no evidence to support routine use of long-term nitrate therapy. There is, however, support for the safety of nitrates during acute myocardial infarction, and they therefore remain a cornerstone in the management of recurrent ischaemia, hypertension and heart failure in this setting.

GP IIb/IIIa antagonists

In recent years it has become apparent that platelets play a central role in acute coronary syndromes. Angioscopy in small numbers of patients has revealed that a white platelet-rich coronary occlusion tends to occur in the setting of unstable angina and subacute closure after coronary angioplasty/stenting. On the other hand, acute myocardial infarction is characterized by an occlusive thrombus which appears red, due to the fibrin-rich clot which surrounds the platelet-rich core. This suggests that platelets play different roles in different coronary syndromes. Furthermore, thrombolysis, while restoring vessel patency, exposes thrombin, which is a potent platelet activator and may account for later vessel re-occlusion.

These insights have stimulated interest in the clinical efficacy of a novel group of drugs that alter platelet function, collectively called the glycoprotein IIb/IIIa inhibitors. Glycoprotein IIb/IIIa is an adhesion molecule which acts as a receptor for fibrinogen and is extremely abundant on platelets (there are about 50 000 receptors on each platelet). A very wide variety of different stimuli can lead to activation of the glycoprotein IIb/IIIa receptor, which then possesses a high affinity for fibrinogen. A platelet-rich thrombus is formed, cross-linked by fibrinogen bridges. Because glycoprotein IIb/IIIa is not expressed on any other cell in the body and represents a necessary and common pathway to platelet aggregation, its inhibition is theoretically an ideal way to tackle clinical syndromes dominated by platelet activation.

Two types of antagonist have been developed. The first is a monoclonal antibody directed at the RGD recognition region of the GP IIb/IIIa molecule. It is called abciximab (also 7E3, Reopro). The second is a group of peptide or peptide-like drugs which mimic the RGD recognition site of fibrinogen and so competitively inhibit its binding to GP IIb/IIIa. These include eptifibatide, tirofiban, lamifiban, xemlifiban and fradifiban.

This section will concentrate on studies that have looked at the treatment of myocardial infarction rather than unstable angina, but Table 8.2 will help put the trials in clinical perspective. The full trial names are given in Table 8.3. The larger of the trials that have

Table 8.2
Trials of glycoprotein IIb/IIIa inhibitors grouped by acute coronary syndrome.

ST elevation
  Primary PTCA
    EPIC
  Fibrinolytic therapy
    TAMI-8, IMPACT-AMI,
    PARADIGM, TIMI 14,
    GUSTO-IV
  Rescue PTCA
    EPIC

No ST elevation
  Urgent PTCA
    EPIC, EPILOG, EPISTENT
  Delayed PTCA
    CAPTURE
  Medical therapy with watchful waiting
    PRISM, PRISM-PLUS, PARAGON,
    PURSUIT, GUSTO-IV

PTCA, percutaneous transluminal coronary angioplasty. Adapted from Braunwald et al.[44]

investigated the treatment of acute myocardial infarction using GP IIb/IIIa blockers are presented in Table 8.4. At present, the majority have evaluated abciximab, and for many the results are available in preliminary form only.

The first two have investigated the use of abciximab in the context of interventional treatment for acute myocardial infarction. The EPIC trial[31] enrolled 2099 patients to assess the potential value of abciximab in 'high-risk' angioplasty. Of this group, 42 were treated by primary angioplasty and 22 by

Table 8.3
Full names of the major trials using glycoprotein IIb/IIIa inhibitors.

	Full name
EPIC [31]	*Evaluation of 7E3 for the Prevention of Ischemic Complications*
RAPPORT [32]	*ReoPro in Acute MI and Primary PTCA Organization and Randomized Trial*
TAMI [33]	*Thrombolysis and Angioplasty in Myocardial Infarction*
TIMI-14 [34]	*Thrombolysis in Myocardial Infarction*
GUSTO-IV	*Global Use of Strategies to Open Occluded Coronary Arteries in Acute Coronary Syndromes*
IMPACT-AMI [35]	*Integrilin to Minimize Platelet Aggregation and Prevent Coronary Thrombosis–Acute Myocardial Infarction*
PARADIGM [36]	*Platelet Aggregation Receptor Antagonist Dose Investigation for Reperfusion Gain in Myocardial Infarction*
EPILOG [37]	*Evaluation in PTCA to Improve Long-Term Outcome with Abciximab GP IIb/IIIa Blockade*
EPISTENT [38]	*Evaluation of Platelet IIb/IIIa Inhibitor for Stenting*
CAPTURE [39]	*c7E3 Fab Antiplatelet Therapy in Unstable Refractory Angina*
PRISM [40]	*The Platelet Receptor Inhibition in Ischaemic Syndrome Management*
PRISM-PLUS [41]	*The Platelet Receptor Inhibition in Ischaemic Syndrome Management in Patients limited by Unstable Angina*
PARAGON [42]	*Platelet IIb/IIIa Antagonism for the Reduction of Acute Coronary Syndrome Events in a Global Organization Network*
PURSUIT [43]	*Platelet IIb/IIIa in Unstable Angina: Receptor Supression Using Integrelin Therapy*

rescue angioplasty. These 64 patients were the focus of a post hoc analysis,[45] and though the numbers were small, there was a large statistically significant benefit, particularly in those patients treated with abciximab bolus followed by a 12-hr infusion (Table 8.4). Enthusiasm for abciximab used in this setting should be tempered by the results of the ReoPro in Acute MI and Primary PTCA Organization and Randomized Trial (RAPPORT). This was a larger trial assessing the use of abciximab (bolus plus 12-h infusion) versus placebo in patients treated by primary angioplasty for acute myocardial infarction. While at 30 days important benefit was observed,[32] the 6-month analysis suggested that this might not be sustained.[46]

Table 8.4
Summary of the trials of glycoprotein IIb/IIIa inhibitors in the treatment of acute myocardial infarction.

Trial	Treatment	Adjunctive Rx	End point	Outcome
EPIC Subgroup n = 64	Placebo versus abciximab bolus versus abciximab bolus + 12-h-infusion	PTCA for AMI (primary and rescue)	Composite of: death + re-MI + re-PTCA + CABG	26.1% versus 21.1% versus 4.5%, p = 0.06 (30 days) 47.8% versus 32.3% versus 4.5%, p = 0.002 (6 months)
RAPPORT n = 483	Abciximab bolus + infusion versus placebo	PTCA for AMI (primary)	Death + re-MI	10.3% versus 4.9%, p = 0.03 (30 days) 28.2% versus 28.1% p = NS (6 months)
TAMI-8 Angiographic subgroup n = 45	Murine 7E3 (different doses at different times) + tPA versus tPA + placebo	Nil	TIMI grade 2 or 3 flow at median 121 h (placebo), 129 h (m7E3)	56% versus 92% (no statistical comparison—see text)
TIMI-14 n = 681	tPA alone or SK (4 dose sizes) + abciximab or tPA (4 dose sizes) + abciximab or abciximab alone	Nil	TIMI-3 flow at 90 min angiography	Abciximab comparable to SK alone, low-dose tPA abciximab promising
GUSTO-IV	Abciximab, tPA or SK	Nil		Recruiting
IMPACT-AMI n = 48 (see text)	Eptifibatide + tPA or placebo + tPA	Nil	TIMI-3 flow at 90 min angiography	66% (highest dose eptifibatide) versus 39%, p = 0.06
PARADIGM n = 150	Lamifiban bolus + infusion versus placebo (in addition to tPA or SK)	Nil	90 min reperfusion assessed by continuous ECG	77% versus 56%, p = 0.02

AMI, acute myocardial infarction; CABG, coronary artery bypass graft; NS, not significant*; PTCA, percutaneous transluminal coronary angioplasty; re-MI, reinfarction; SK, streptokinase; TIMI, thrombolysis in myocardial infarction; *PA, *tissue plasminogen activator.

There has also been interest in the use of IIb/IIIa inhibitors to potentiate the effects of thrombolytic therapy in the pharmacological treatment of myocardial infarction. In 1993 the results of the TAMI-8 pilot study were published. This was the first assessment of a glycoprotein IIb/IIIa antagonist in combination with thrombolytic therapy for acute myocardial infarction. It was a dose escalation and timing trial using murine 7E3 (an early non-chimeric form of abciximab) in conjunction with tPA. Escalating boluses of m7E3 were given at 15 h after thrombolysis in some patients, others received escalating doses at 6 h, and others at 3 h after thrombolysis. This complexity made definitive conclusions about efficacy difficult to draw (it was designed as a safety and physiological activity pilot), but in the angiographic sub-study comparing all the 37 patients who received m7E3 with the nine receiving placebo, there was evidence of improved TIMI grade 2 or 3 flow.[33]

More recently, the results of the TIMI-14 study have been presented.[34] This complex dose-ranging study randomized 681 patients suffering acute myocardial infarction to four groups (see Table 8.4). The provisional findings were that abciximab alone resulted in TIMI grade 3 flow of 32% (similar to streptokinase (SK) alone in earlier studies). The combination of reduced-dose thrombolytic plus abciximab enhanced TIMI grade 3 flow. The price for this benefit (certainly with SK plus abciximab) was an increased risk of haemorrhagic complications. The combination of reduced-dose tPA plus abciximab seemed a promising alternative to full-dose accelerated tPA alone. GUSTO-IV, which is currently recruiting, may clarify some of the questions raised by TIMI-14.

There are also a number of studies on the efficacy of the peptide and peptide-like GP IIb/IIIa inhibitors. Two have reported at the time of writing. Eptifibatide in combination with tPA was evaluated in IMPACT-AMI.[35] The first part of this study was a dose-ranging assessment with 132 patients. Another 48 were then randomized to compare the highest epifibatide dose (plus tPA) with placebo (plus tPA). Though the primary end-point of TIMI grade 3 angiographic patency was improved in the eptifibatide-treated group, the composite end-point of in-hospital death, reinfarction, stroke, revascularization, new heart failure or pulmonary oedema was unaltered by the drug. In PARADIGM, lamifiban was used as an adjunct to tPA or SK. The preliminary results showed improved 90-min infarct-related artery patency as judged by continuous ECG monitoring, but the final results have not yet been published.[36]

In conclusion, it can be seen that there are currently many unanswered questions about the role of these drugs in the management of acute myocardial infarction. In the context of other trials assessing their use in the setting of unstable coronary syndromes, it is likely that at least abciximab will have an important role in combination with interventional techniques. When they are used as an adjunct to thrombolysis, it seems likely that coronary patency rates can be improved, but it is not yet clear whether this will be at the cost of prohibitive haemorrhagic complications. There also appear to be differences in the efficacy of the agents under investigation. Abciximab appears to be more potent than the small RGD mimetics. The reason for this is unclear, but IIb/IIIa binding by these agents in the absence of fibrinogen may not simply block platelet aggregation, because there is evidence of internal cellular signalling. The problem may be that they act as partial agonists.

ACE inhibitors

In the immediate aftermath of a myocardial infarction, ventricular cavity dilatation and stimulation of neurohumoral systems maintain cardiac output. Dilatation improves cardiac output by a Frank–Starling mechanism, and renin–angiotensin and adrenosympathetic drives result in inotropic stimulation of the remaining functional myocardium, peripheral vasoconstriction and salt and water retention. After about 3 days, if left ventricular function is not significantly damaged, neurohumoral activation wanes. If there is significant dysfunction, then the activation persists. The damaged muscle thins, expands and becomes fibrotic. The remaining myocardium undergoes hypertrophy. Approximately a third of infarct survivors develop dilatation, and one-third no change, and in the final third ventricular volumes improve as myocardium recovers from stunning. Catecholamines and angiotensin, while mediating beneficial compensatory effects, have also been implicated in myocyte necrosis in viable regions. It is probably by altering the balance between remodelling and necrosis that ACE inhibitors benefit some patients immediately after infarction.

There have been eight important trials that have clarified the role of ACE inhibitors in patients suffering acute myocardial infarction (Tables 8.5 and 8.6). Only one of these trials (CONSENSUS-II[47]) showed a trend to a harmful effect. It was the only trial to use intravenous administration, and was stopped early after concerns about hypotension, particularly among the elderly, and because of a 10% increase in mortality in the treated arm. There were wide confidence limits (7% benefit to 29% harm). All other studies have used oral agents and demonstrated benefit. These trials have used a variety of drugs at differing doses. The timing of administration has varied, as has the patient population randomized.

Table 8.5
Full names of the trials of angiotensin-converting enzyme inhibitors used at the time of acute myocardial infarction.

	Full name
CONSENUS[47]	Cooperative New Scandinavian Enalapril Survival Study
AIRE[48]	Acute Infarction Ramipril Efficacy
SMILE[49]	Survival of Myocardial Infarction Long-Term Evaluation
TRACE[50]	Trandolapril Cardiac Evaluation
ISIS-4[30]	International Study of Infarct Survival
GISSI-3[29]	Gruppo Italiano per lo Studio della Sopravvivenza nell'infarto Miocardico
CCS[51]	Chinese Cardiac Study
SAVE[52]	Survival And Ventricular Enlargement trial

Table 8.6
Summary of the trials of angiotensin-converting enzyme inhibitors used at the time of acute myocardial infarction.

Trial	N	Patient characteristics	Time between AMI and treatment	Drug and target dose	End point time	Mortality (%) Placebo v treatment	p value
Selective for ↓LV							
AIRE	2006	Clinical failure	3 to 10 days	Ramipril 5 mg bd	mean 15 months	17 v 23	0.002
SMILE	1556	Anterior AMI and no lysis	<24 hours	Zofenopril 30 mg bd	12 months	10 v 14	0.01
TRACE	1749	Echo	3 to 7 days	Trandolapril 4 mg od	24–50 months	34.7 v 42.3	0.001
SAVE	2231	Radionuclide ventriculogram	3 to 16 days	Captopril 50 mg tds	mean 42 months	20 v 25	0.019
Unselective							
CONSENSUS II	6090		<24 hours	Enalapril iv then po	6 months	10.2 v 11	NS
ISIS-4	58050		<24 hours	Captopril 50 mg tds	5 weeks	7.19 v 7.69	0.02
GISSI-3	19394		<24 hours	Lisinopril 10 mg od	6 weeks	7.1 v 6.3	0.03
CCS	13634		<36 hours	Captopril 12.5 mg tds	4 weeks	9.59 v 9.05	NS

AMI = acute myocardial infarction, ↓LV = impaired left ventricular function; NS = not significant.

The greatest benefits have been observed when patients with impaired systolic function have been selected for treatment. This was judged clinically in AIRE,[48] on the basis of an anterior infarction and contraindication to thrombolysis in SMILE,[49] by measuring echo ejection fraction in TRACE,[50] and by radionuclide scans in SAVE.[52] In trials where treatment was started irrespective of left ventricular function (GISSI-3,[29] ISIS-4,[30] CCS[51]), the benefit has been modest (Table 8.5). If estimates of additional lifespan are calculated from the shift in survival curves, the unselected trials appear to deliver a gain of about 1 week, while those selecting patients for impaired left ventricular function deliver a gain of a few months. In addition to reduced mortality, these studies have all demonstrated a reduction in morbidity from heart failure as judged, for example, by hospital admissions.

The decision about whether to give ACE inhibitors to all presenting with acute myocardial infarction (as in GISSI-3, ISIS-4 and CCS), or to wait a few days to allow left ventricular dysfunction to become evident, cannot be made on the basis of the current trials. These strategies have not been directly compared (and probably never will be), so one can only speculate as to which is the most appropriate. The major part of the beneficial effect in the non-selective trials did occur in the first 24 h, suggesting that perhaps all should receive treatment. Nevertheless, this

benefit at 24 h was not statistically significant. Furthermore, the sort of difference in benefit observed between the non-selective and selective trials is compatible with the hypothesis that the overall benefit seen in the unselective trials is due to benefit in the subgroup with left ventricular dysfunction, diluted by no benefit (or even a deleterious effect) in those without significant left ventricular dysfunction.[50] An alternative strategy would be to start all patients with acute myocardial infarction on ACE inhibitors, but discontinue the drug in those patients who later show no evidence of left ventricular dysfunction, either after the first day or before discharge.[53]

If a non-selected approach to treatment is adopted, then there are no data supporting therapy for more than 5 or 6 weeks. The selective trials all continued therapy long term, and survival curves continued to separate. In the context of the known beneficial effects of these drugs in patients with chronic heart failure, long-term treatment is appropriate.

In conclusion, there are good data supporting the beneficial effects of ACE inhibitors started soon after acute myocardial infarction. A strategy of starting treatment in those patients with evidence of left ventricular dysfunction after a few days seems well supported by available evidence. It seems likely that those with impaired left ventricular function have the most to gain both from a reduction in mortality and a reduction in heart failure morbidity, and this group should remain on long-term therapy.

References

1. Braunwald E, Muller JE, Kloner RA, Maroko PR, Role of beta-adrenergic blockade in the therapy of patients with myocardial infarction, *Am J Med* 1983; 74: 113–23.

2. The Norwegian Multicenter Study Group, Timolol-induced reduction in mortality and reinfarction in patients surviving acute myocardial infarction, *N Engl J Med* 1981; 304: 801–7.

3. Beta-Blocker Heart Attack Trial Research Group, A randomized trial of propranolol in patients with acute myocardial infarction. I. Mortality results, *JAMA* 1982; 247: 1707–14.

4. Hjalmarson A, Elmfeldt D, Herlitz J et al, Effect on mortality of metoprolol in acute myocardial infarction: a double blind randomised trial, *Lancet* 1981; ii: 823–7.

5. The MIAMI Trial Research Group, Metoprolol in acute myocardial infarction. Mortality, *Am J Cardiol* 1985; 56: 15G–22G.

6. ISIS-1 (First International Study of Infarct Survival) Collaborative Group, Randomized trial of intravenous atenolol among 16 027 cases of suspected acute myocardial infarction: ISIS-1, *Lancet* 1986; ii: 57–66.

7. Herlitz J, Waagstein F, Lindqvist J et al, Effect of metoprolol on the prognosis for patients with suspected acute myocardial infarction and indirect signs of congestive heart failure (a subgroup analysis of the Goteborg Metoprolol Trial), *Am J Cardiol* 1997; 80: 40J–4J.

8. ISIS-1 (First International Study of Infarct Survival) Collaborative Group, Mechanisms for the early mortality reduction produced by beta-blockade started early in acute myocardial infarction: ISIS-1 (published erratum appears in *Lancet* 1988; 30(2):292), *Lancet* 1988; 1: 921–3.

9. Pollak H, Nobis H, Mlczoch J, Frequency of left ventricular free wall rupture complicating acute myocardial infarction since the advent of thrombolysis, *Am J Cardiol* 1994; 74: 184–6.

10. Becker RC, Charlesworth A, Wilcox RG et al, Cardiac rupture associated with thrombolytic therapy: impact of time to treatment in the Late Assessment of Thrombolytic Efficacy (LATE) study, *J Am Coll Cardiol* 1995; 25: 1063–8.

11. Hammerman H, Kloner RA, Briggs LL, Braunwald E, Enhancement of salvage of reperfused myocardium by early beta-adrenergic blockade (timolol), *J Am Coll Cardiol* 1984; 3: 1438–43.

12. Roberts R, Rogers WJ, Mueller HS et al, Immediate versus deferred beta-blockade following thrombolytic therapy in patients with acute myocardial infarction. Results of the Thrombolysis in Myocardial Infarction (TIMI) II-B Study, *Circulation* 1991; 83: 422–37.

13. Basu S, Senior R, Raval U et al, Beneficial effects of intravenous and oral carvedilol treatment in acute myocardial infarction. A placebo-controlled, randomized trial, *Circulation* 1997; 96: 183–91.

14. Kendall MJ, Clinical relevance of pharmacokinetic differences between beta blockers, *Am J Cardiol* 1997; 80: 15J–19J.

15. Julian DG, Prescott RJ, Jackson FS, Szekely P, Controlled trial of sotalol for one year after

myocardial infarction, *Lancet* 1982; **1:** 1142–7.

16. Gruppo Italiano per lo Studio della Sopravvivenza nell'Infarto Miocardico, GISSI-2: a factorial randomised trial of alteplase versus streptokinase and heparin versus no heparin among 12,490 patients with acute myocardial infarction, *Lancet* 1990; **336:** 65–71.

17. Mafrici A, Mauri F, Maggioni AP et al, Atenolol i.v. in the acute phase of AMI: the indications, contraindications and interactions with thrombolytic drugs in the GISSI-2 study, *G Ital di Cardiol* 1995; **25:** 353–64.

18. Wilcox RG, Hampton JR, Banks DC et al, Trial of early nifedipine in acute myocardial infarction: the Trent study, *Br Med J* 1994; **1986:** 1204–8.

19. Sirnes PA, Overskeid K, Pedersen TR et al, Evolution of infarct size during the early use of nifedipine in patients with acute myocardial infarction: the Norwegian Nifedipine Multicenter Trial, *Circulation* 1984; **70:** 638–44.

20. Goldbourt U, Behar S, Reicher-Reiss H et al, Early administration of nifedipine in suspected acute myocardial infarction. The Secondary Prevention Reinfarction Israel Nifedipine Trial 2 Study, *Arch Intern Med* 1993; **153:** 345–53.

21. Muller JE, Morrison J, Stone PH et al, Nifedipine therapy for patients with threatened and acute myocardial infarction: a randomized, double-blind, placebo-controlled comparison, *Circulation* 1984; **69:** 740–7.

22. The Danish Study Group on Verapamil in Myocardial Infarction, Verapamil in acute myocardial infarction, *Eur Heart J* 1984; **5:** 516–28.

23. The Danish Verapamil Infarction Trial II—DAVIT II, Effect of verapamil on mortality and major events after acute myocardial infarction, *Am J Cardiol* 1990; **66:** 779–85.

24. The Multicenter Diltiazem Postinfarction Trial Research Group, The effect of diltiazem on mortality and reinfarction after myocardial infarction, *N Engl J Med* 1988; **319:** 385–92.

25. Gibson RS, Boden WE, Theroux P et al, Diltiazem and reinfarction in patients with non-Q-wave myocardial infarction, *N Engl J Med* 1986; **315:** 423–9.

26. Boden WE, Scheldewaert R, Walters EG et al, Design of a placebo-controlled clinical trial of long-acting diltiazem and aspirin versus aspirin alone in patients receiving thrombolysis with a first acute myocardial infarction. Incomplete Infarction Trial of European Research Collaborators Evaluating Prognosis Post-Thrombolysis (diltiazem) (INTERCEPT) Research Group, *Am J Cardiol* 1995; **75:** 1120–3.

27. Jugdutt BI, Warnica JW, Intravenous nitroglycerin therapy to limit myocardial infarct size, expansion, and complications. Effect of timing, dosage, and infarct location, *Circulation* 1988; **78:** 906–919 (published erratum appears in *Circulation 1989;* 79(5): 1151.

28. Yusuf S, Collins R, MacMahon S, Peto R, Effect of intravenous nitrates on mortality in acute myocardial infarction: an overview of the randomised trials, *Lancet* 1988; **1:** 1088–92.

29. Gruppo Italiano per lo Studio della Sopravvivenza nell'infarto Miocardico, GISSI-3: effects of lisinopril and transdermal glyceryl trinitrate singly and together on 6-week mortality and ventricular function after acute myocardial infarction, *Lancet* 1994; **343:** 1115–22.

30. ISIS-4 (Fourth International Study of Infarct Survival) Collaborative Group, ISIS-4: a randomised factorial trial assessing early oral captopril, oral mononitrate, and intravenous magnesium sulphate in 58,050 patients with suspected acute myocardial infarction, *Lancet* 1995; **345**: 669–85.

31. The EPIC Investigators, Use of a monoclonal antibody directed against the platelet glycoprotein IIb/IIIa receptor in high-risk coronary angioplasty. The EPIC Investigation, *N Engl J Med* 1994; **330**: 956–61.

32. Brener SJ, Barr LA, Cohen ED et al, Abciximab reduces urgent target vessel revascularization at 30 days after primary angioplasty, independently of acute angiographic results. The RAPPORT Trial, *J Am Coll Cardiol* 1998; **31**(suppl A): 54A.

33. Kleiman NS, Ohman EM, Califf RM et al, Profound inhibition of platelet aggregation with monoclonal antibody 7E3 Fab after thrombolytic therapy. Results of the Thrombolysis and Angioplasty in Myocardial Infarction (TAMI) 8 Pilot Study, *J Am Coll Cardiol* 1993; **22**: 381–9.

34. Antman EM, Giugliano RP, McCabe CH et al, Abciximab (ReoPrp) potentiates thrombolysis in ST elevation myocardial infarction: results of TIMI 14 trial, *J Am Coll Cardiol* 1998; **31**(suppl A): 191A (abstract).

35. Ohman EM, Kleiman NS, Gacioch G et al, Combined accelerated tissue-plasminogen activator and platelet glycoprotein IIb/IIIa integrin receptor blockade with Integrilin in acute myocardial infarction. Results of a randomized, placebo-controlled, dose-ranging trial. IMPACT-AMI Investigators, *Circulation* 1997; **95**: 846–54.

36. Moliterno DJ, Krucoff MW, Armstrong PW et al, More complete and stable reperfusion with platelet iib/iiia antagonism plus thrombolysis for AMI: The PARADIGM Trial, *Circulation* 1996; **94**: I-553 (abstract).

37. The EPILOG Investigators, Platelet glycoprotein IIb/IIIa receptor blockade and low-dose heparin during percutaneous coronary revascularization, *N Engl J Med* 1997; **336**: 1689–96.

38. The EPISTENT Investigators, Randomised placebo-controlled and balloon-angioplasty controlled trial to assess safety of coronary stenting with the use of platelet glycoprotein-IIb/IIIa blockade, *Lancet* 1998; **352**: 87–92.

39. The CAPTURE Investigators, Randomised placebo-controlled trial of abciximab before and during coronary intervention in refractory unstable angina: the CAPTURE Study, *Lancet* 1997; **349**: 1429–35 (published erratum appears in *Lancet* 1997; **6**(350): 744).

40. The PRISM Study Investigators, A comparison of aspirin plus tirofiban with aspirin plus heparin for unstable angina, *N Engl J Med* 1998; **338**: 1498–505.

41. The PRISM-PLUS Study Investigators, Inhibition of the platelet glycoprotein IIb/IIIa receptor with tirofiban in unstable angina and non-Q-wave myocardial infarction, *N Engl J Med* 1998; **338**: 1488–97.

42. The PARAGON Investigators, International, randomized, controlled trial of lamifiban (a platelet glycoprotein IIb/IIIa inhibitor), heparin, or both in unstable angina, Platelet IIb/IIIa, *Circulation* 1998; **97**: 2386–95.

43. Harrington RA, Design and methodology of the PURSUIT trial: evaluating eptifibatide for acute ischemic coronary syndromes. Platelet glycoprotein IIb-IIIa in unstable angina: receptor suppression using integrilin therapy, *Am Heart J* 1997; **80**: 34B–8B.

44. Braunwald E, Maseri A, Armstrong PW et al, Rationale and clinical evidence for the use of GP IIb/IIIa inhibitors in acute coronary syndromes, *Eur Heart J* 1998; **19**(suppl D):D22–30.

45. Lefkovits J, Ivanhoe RJ, Califf RM et al, Effects of platelet glycoprotein IIb/IIIa receptor blockade by a chimeric monoclonal antibody (abciximab) on acute and six-month outcomes after percutaneous transluminal coronary angioplasty for acute myocardial infarction. EPIC investigators, *Am J Cardiol* 1996; **77**: 1045–1051.

46. Brener SJ, Barr LA, Burchenal J et al, A randomized placebo controlled trial of abciximab with primary angioplasty for acute MI: the RAPPORT trial, *Circulation* 1998; **96**(suppl I): I473 (abstract).

47. Swedberg K, Held P, Kjekshus J et al, Effects of the early administration of enalapril on mortality in patients with acute myocardial infarction. Results of the Cooperative New Scandinavian Enalapril Survival Study II (CONSENSUS II), *N Engl J Med* 1992; **327**: 678–84.

48. The Acute Infarction Ramipril Efficacy (AIRE) Study Investigators, Effect of ramipril on mortality and morbidity of survivors of acute myocardial infarction with clinical evidence of heart failure, *Lancet* 1993; **342**: 821–8.

49. Ambrosioni E, Borghi C, Magnani B, The effect of the angiotensin-converting-enzyme inhibitor zofenopril on mortality and morbidity after anterior myocardial infarction. The Survival of Myocardial Infarction Long-Term Evaluation (SMILE) Study Investigators, *N Engl J Med* 1995; **332**: 80–5.

50. Kober L, Torp-Pedersen C, Carlsen JE et al, A clinical trial of the angiotensin-converting-enzyme inhibitor trandolapril in patients with left ventricular dysfunction after myocardial infarction. Trandolapril Cardiac Evaluation (TRACE) Study Group, *N Engl J Med* 1995; **333**: 1670–6.

51. Oral captopril versus placebo among 13,634 patients with suspected acute myocardial infarction: interim report from the Chinese Cardiac Study (CCS-1), *Lancet* 1995; **345**: 686–7.

52. Pfeffer MA, Braunwald E, Moye LA et al, Effect of captopril on mortality and morbidity in patients with left ventricular dysfunction after myocardial infarction. Results of the survival and ventricular enlargement trial. The SAVE Investigators, *N Engl J Med* 1992; **327**: 669–77.

53. Coats AJS, ACE inhibitors after myocardial infarction: selection and treatment for all, *Br Heart J* 1995; **73**: 395–6.

Coronary angioplasty and stenting

Adrian Brodison and Anoop Chauhan

9

Angioplasty in myocardial infarction

The search for the 'gold standard' treatment for acute myocardial infarction (AMI) has produced, without doubt, the greatest volume of research and study of any area of medicine in the modern era–justifiably so for the condition which is still, despite all the advances, the largest single cause of mortality in the Western world.

Mortality from AMI has been falling steadily for most of this century, and according to some estimates[1,2] about 40% of the fall in mortality until the late 1980s was due to coronary care units, pre-hospital resuscitation and newer medical treatments. It is the latter which has contributed to the continued decline in case fatality rates and to which the rest of this chapter will refer.

The use of aspirin,[3] beta-blockers[4] and, more latterly, angiotensin inhibitors[5] has contributed to the reduction in mortality after AMI, but none of these measures actually addresses the underlying cause of the AMI, namely thrombosis. Restoration of normal bloodflow in an infarct-related coronary artery is the 'holy grail' of modern cardiology. The earliest attempts at thrombus dissolution using intravenous thrombolytic agents brought significant reductions in mortality of 20–30%.[3,6,7] More recently, the use of the more specific agent recombinant tissue plasminogen activator (r-tPA) when used in an 'accelerated' approach has produced further benefits, especially in high-risk groups, when compared with streptokinase. The GUSTO 1 trial showed that anterior myocardial infarction had a greater benefit in terms of mortality reduction from r-tPA than streptokinase (8.6% versus 10.5%). The comparable rates for inferior myocardial infarction were 4.7% versus 5.7%, respectively.[8] Despite these improvements, angiographic sub-studies have shown that reperfusion rates are less. Restoration of normal Thrombolysis In Myocardial Infarction (TIMI 3) flow in the infarct-related artery at 90 min after commencement of thrombolytic therapy was found in 29–54%.[7,9] This result was maintained 5–7 days later, with TIMI 3 flow rates of 51–58%. Initially, indirect evidence from experimental studies suggested that an 'open' infarct-related vessel confers a better outcome irrespective of any myocardial salvage.[10] The Western Washington trial of intracoronary streptokinase showed that patients with restoration of vessel patency had significantly improved long-term prognosis when compared to those with partial or no

reperfusion, without any improvement in myocardial function.[11] These observations lead to the logical conclusion that thrombolysis should be followed by immediate coronary angiography and angioplasty if appropriate. Further support for an invasive approach was provided by Serruys et al, when it was found that 70% of infarct-related vessels still had significant stenosis after thrombolysis.[12] A severe residual stenosis also correlates with a high rate of early reocclusion.[13] Early angiography gave the added benefit of accurately defining coronary anatomy allowing early triage to surgery.

One of the major questions which has to be answered is on whom, if any, should coronary intervention be performed following thrombolysis. The approaches vary between angioplasty in those with satisfactory reperfusion but residual stenosis, restricting intervention to those with evidence of reduced perfusion (less than TIMI grade 3), or dealing only with those who have failed to reperfuse, so-called 'rescue angioplasty'. The other obvious question is when should the timing of this intervention take place, immediately or shortly after the initiating or completion of thrombolysis, after some hours, after a few days, or only if the patient has further evidence of cardiac ischaemia.

Regrettably, much of the work done in this area has involved trials which have not been fully randomized, and the results have often been somewhat biased by the understandable desire of the interventional cardiologist not to leave the patient with an artery with insufficient antegrade bloodflow. However, much information has now been gained and conclusions can be drawn.

Thrombolysis followed by angioplasty

There was initial optimism when two trials were published showing an apparent benefit from early angioplasty following either intracoronary or intravenous streptokinase.[14,15] This led to the organization of larger-scale trials to confirm these results.

The European Co-operative Study Group Trial of r-tPA and conservative therapy versus r-tPA and immediate angioplasty randomized patients with TIMI grade 0 or 1, and patients with a higher TIMI grade but with a residual stenosis of >60% in the infarct-related vessel.[16] The trial was terminated early after the ethical review committee found that there was no difference in the primary end-points of infarct size and left ventricular function and a non-significant trend towards increased mortality in the invasive group (15 versus 6 deaths). In fairness to the trial, further analysis revealed that of the 15 patients who died, only 11 had angioplasty attempted and it had been successful in seven (Table 9.1). These discouraging results were supported by the

Table 9.1
Results of rescue PTCA and conservative treatment in failed thrombolysis.

	Number	PTCA	Success rate (%)	Reocclusion (%)	Mortality, PTCA(%)	Mortality, conservative treatment (%)
ECSG[16]	367	183[a]	92	–	8.2	3.3
TAMI 1–5[20]	776	169	–	–	5.9	4.6
CORAMI[23]	72	72	92	7	4	–
ELLIS[22]	151	92	92	8	5.1	9.6[b]
GUSTO I[21]	214	214	90	12	8.6	5.2

CORAMI, Cohort of Rescue Angioplasty in Myocardial Infarction; ECSG, European Co-operative Study Group; ELLIS, Ellis SG, GUSTO I, Global Utilisation of Strategies To open Occluded coronary arteries angiographic substudy; TAMI 1–5, Review of the first five Thrombolysis and Angioplasty in Myocardial Infarction trials; PTCA, percutaneous transluminal coronary angioplasty. Success was generally defined as restoration of TIMI grade 2–3 and residual stenosis <50%. [a]Only 168 of those randomized had PTCA performed; [b]p < 0.05.

similar TIMI IIA, where there were higher rates of bypass surgery and bleeding complications in the invasive group.[17]

A slightly different approach was adopted in the Thrombolysis and Angioplasty in Myocardial Infarction (TAMI) 1 trial, where the question addressed was, having achieved coronary artery patency, how best this could be maintained. TAMI 1 randomized patients with patent infarct vessels and suitable anatomy to immediate versus deferred angioplasty.[18,19] This showed a higher mortality, requirement for emergency coronary artery bypass surgery and requirement for transfusion in the angioplasty group, with no difference in ejection fraction or reocclusion between the two groups. However, the reocclusion rate was still worryingly high at 29%.

The TAMI group of investigators have gone on to perform a series of further trials looking at various thrombolytic regimens and to specifically address the issue of rescue angioplasty. In a review of the first five TAMI trials, 169 of 776 patients had infarct-related vessels achieve patency by angioplasty after failed thrombolysis, the remainder having achieved patency by thrombolysis.[20] When the thrombolysis and angioplasty patency groups were compared, the former had higher acute and 7–10-day left ventricular ejection fractions and greater infarct zone recovery,

and reocclusion was less. In-hospital mortality rates were shown to be similar, and long-term mortality rates were also similar (Table 9.1).

In the largest trial of 'rescue' angioplasty[21] during the GUSTO angiographic sub-study, the investigators reported angiographic success in 90% of patients, a figure which is similar to that achieved in other groups.[22–24] The main outcome was the marked difference in 30-day mortality in those patients in whom rescue angioplasty was unsuccessful (30.4%), compared to successful rescue (8.6%) and to successful thrombolysis (5.2%). This has also been observed by other workers.[25] Prior to this study it was believed that complication rates after rescue PTCA are high,[17,26] but here there was no significant increase in major bleeding, surgical repair of vascular access site, emergency coronary artery bypass graft surgery (CABG) or stroke. It must be stressed that rescue attempts were not randomized and therefore only give inferential information regarding the clinical usefulness of this procedure. Ellis' randomized trial has suggested that there may be a borderline significant difference in the combined endpoint of death or severe heart failure in favour of rescue angioplasty (Table 9.1).[22] However, only exercise, and not resting, left ventricular ejection fraction was significantly improved (43% versus 38%, $p = 0.04$).

From the available information, it can be

suggested that angioplasty following thrombolysis has limited use and then only in selected subgroups, specifically those in whom thrombolysis has failed. The difficulty arises in accurately identifying those patients in whom thrombolysis has failed. The reason why there is no benefit in left ventricular function or long-term mortality may be the delay in reperfusion or the relatively high reocclusion rates. In patients who have been thrombolysed, it has been suggested that a policy of 'watchful waiting' may be best, with intervention being directed towards those who have evidence of ongoing or recurrent ischaemia.[27]

An issue which has not yet been addressed is whether there are any alternatives to rescue angioplasty or conservative treatment when thrombolysis has failed. Hopefully, the answer will come from the Rescue Angioplasty versus Conservative treatment or repeat Thrombolysis (REACT) trial. This trial, which is due to start enrolling patients soon, is comparing the outcome in patients with failed thrombolysis when they are randomized to rescue angioplasty, further thrombolysis or conservative treatment (intravenous heparin for 24 h). This trial could potentially have significant implications regarding the provision of interventional facilities and transfer of patients to these facilities, although it will be some time before results are available (December 2001).

Primary angioplasty versus thrombolysis

To the limitations of thrombolysis mentioned previously need to be added the contraindications to thrombolysis, such as recent stroke, surgery or trauma and the risk of stroke and bleeding complications as a result of the therapy of about 1%.[9,28] It would seem logical, therefore, to investigate a treatment for AMI which avoids the need for thrombolytic therapy.

The primary angioplasty debate was commenced by the simultaneous publication of three trials in 1993 comparing primary angioplasty with thrombolytic therapy.[29–31] Each of these trials comprised relatively small numbers, making definite conclusions regarding the definitive end-point of death difficult to arrive at. However, two of the trials[29,30] did reach positive conclusions regarding the benefits of the procedure. Grines' group[29] showed that percutaneous transluminal coronary angioplasty (PTCA) produced significant reductions in in-hospital mortality in a subgroup judged to be 'not low risk'. The rates of recurrent ischaemia, haemorrhagic strokes, and non-fatal reinfarction and death were also significantly reduced in the primary PTCA group. Zijlstra's group[30] had the advantage of angiographic assessment in both arms of the study, and concluded that higher rates of patency were shown in the angioplasty group. Repeat angiography in the PTCA group at 3 months showed a patency rate of 91% versus 68% patency in the streptokinase group at a not strictly comparable 3-week angiogram ($p = 0.001$). They also found lower rates of reinfarction and unstable angina, less severe residual stenotic lesion and marginally better left ventricular ejection fractions in the angioplasty group. This study has had further patients enrolled in an extension to the original study.[32] The combined results have shown significant reductions in in-hospital mortality and reinfarction and more impressive improvements in left ventricular ejection fraction in the angioplasty group. Gibbons' group[31] found no significant differences in the degree of myocardial salvage or in any of the other variables mentioned in the other studies. The reason

for this apparent difference in results may be easily explained. All three studies had similarly high success rates with angioplasty (92–98%).

Since the publication of these studies, there have been many more trials of primary angioplasty compared to thrombolytic therapy. The problem of small patient numbers has to some extent been circumvented by a comprehensive meta-analysis[33] of all the randomized studies, comparing primary angioplasty with thrombolysis up to the end of 1997 (Table 9.2).[25,29–32,34–38] It has to be acknowledged that there are limitations in combining data from many different studies with different inclusion criteria, therapy protocols and clinical end-points. However, the subject is almost unique, in that, despite differences, the opening of an

Table 9.2
Combined meta-analysis results for primary PTCA versus thrombolysis.

	Primary PTCA	Thrombolysis	p value
Number randomized	1290	1316	–
Time to treatment (min)	90	57	<0.001
Total mortality (%)	4.4	6.5	0.02
Total mortality and non-fatal reinfarction (%)	7.2	11.9	<0.001
Major bleeding (%)	8.8	8.4	0.74
Total stroke (%)	0.7	2.0	<0.001

End of study was used as the time of reporting of end-points, as 30-day results were not quoted for each study.

occluded artery by a balloon in the setting of a myocardial infarct is a remarkably similar procedure irrespective of the study protocol. The review subdivided the different thrombolytic regimens into those using streptokinase, a 3–4-h infusion of tPA or a 4-h infusion of alteplase, and those using a 90-min 'accelerated' infusion of tPA, to prevent the previously published better results with tPA[8] being negatively affected by being grouped with streptokinase. In all, 2606 patients were randomized, 1316 received thrombolytic therapy, of whom 307 received streptokinase, 300 received 3–4-h tPA or duteplase, and 709 received 'accelerated' tPA. Not surprisingly in a trial setting, there was only a 26-min delay on average to treatment by angioplasty when compared to thrombolysis.

The overall risk of death was significantly reduced in favour of PTCA, although each thrombolytic subgroup was not large enough by itself to produce a significant reduction (Table 9.2). The combined meta-analysis results showed that the risk of death was 4.4% in the PTCA group and 6.5% in the thrombolytic group. This translates into an additional 21 lives per 1000 patients treated. An examination of the combined end-points of death or non-fatal reinfarction showed each subgroup to have a significant reduction in favour of PTCA, as did the meta-analysis of all the subgroups (7.2% versus 11.9%). This

represents 46 fewer events per 1000 patients treated. There was a trend for the 'accelerated' tPA treatment group to be better than the other thrombolytic regimens, but this did not reach significance levels. Total stroke rates were significantly better in the combined data for PTCA (0.7% versus 2.0%), as was the rate of haemorrhagic stroke (0.1% versus 1.1%). This difference was most marked in the 'accelerated' tPA trials. The risk of major bleeding was similar between all groups, with 8.8% of PTCA patients and 8.4% of thrombolytic patients having at least one major bleeding episode. One of the criticisms of this meta-analysis is the relatively large effect of a single study, the GUSTO IIB study,[25] which enrolled more patients (1138) than any of the others. The authors of the meta-analysis did perform tests of heterogeneity and compared this trial with the others. They found that there was evidence of heterogeneity between the trials and that in the GUSTO IIB trial it was only the difference in the composite end-point of death, non-fatal reinfarction and non-fatal disabling stroke which reached significance levels, with each of the end-points themselves producing non-significant reductions.

Should these results make us all want to throw away our syringes of thrombolytic agents and reach for our angioplasty balloons? Aside from the lack of availability of cardiac catheterization facilities in most hospitals, there are many issues which still need to be investigated. Are the beneficial effects of PTCA maintained for longer than the 30-day follow-up used in most trials? Evidence from the GUSTO IIB trial,[25] which included 6-month follow-up, suggested that there was no difference in end-points after this time. This finding may have been a result of a relatively high rate of reocclusion which has been noted in serial angiographic studies.[39] Should the use of angioplasty be reserved for those patients judged to be at higher risk? Zijlstra's study[32] specifically looked at 'low-risk' patients, who had no contraindication to thrombolytic therapy, Killip class <2 and non-extensive infarction by ECG criteria. The conclusions were that the primary end-point of death, non-fatal reinfarction and stroke were significantly lower in the angioplasty arm, although the numbers randomized were small. Further studies are required before conclusive recommendations in this area can be adopted.

Many patients are considered ineligible for thrombolytic therapy due to the number of contraindications to this therapy. Paradoxically, it is often this group of patients who have most to gain from reperfusion therapy. They are more likely to be female, older, and have had previous infarcts, multivessel disease, lower ejection fraction, and higher in-hospital mortality (18.7% versus 3.9%, $p < 0.001$).[40] Primary PTCA can

often be performed in these patients, who would otherwise be denied potentially life-saving therapy. There is a significant increase in procedure-related mortality due to comorbid disease when compared to thrombolytic-eligible patients (14% versus 3%).[41] However, when the strict eligibility criteria of TIMI IIB were applied, better early and late results were achieved with PTCA versus tPA (Table 9.3).[42]

Can results from these trials, which have generally been performed in centres with high levels of expertise and dedication to provision of primary angioplasty facilities, be extrapolated to the wider population of hospitals? Primary angioplasty is a more technically demanding procedure than elective angioplasty and is associated with an operator-dependent morbidity and mortality that varies with the skill and experience of that operator.[43] There has also been a suggestion that primary angioplasty procedures should be carried out in centres without surgical backup, thereby potentially allowing more hospitals to offer this service.[44] In the trials mentioned above, significant numbers of patients assigned to angioplasty actually had CABG performed instead, and of those undergoing angioplasty, generally more required CABG than those in the thrombolysis arm. Given that the trials were generally analysed on an 'intention-to-treat' basis and that the CABG patients generally had good results, this may

Table 9.3
PTCA versus tPA for acute myocardial infarction.

	Lytic eligible[a]			Lytic ineligible[a]		
	PTCA	**tPA**	**p-value**	**PTCA**	**tPA**	**p-value**
Number	127	117	–	68	83	–
In-hospital death (%)	2.4	1.7	NS	2.9	13.2	0.015
In-hospital death or re-MI (%)	5.5	9.4	NS	4.4	15.7	0.025
6-month death (%)	3.9	1.7	NS	2.9	15.7	0.009
6-month death or re-MI (%)	8.7	12.8	NS	7.3	22.9	0.009

[a]Lytic eligibility based on TIMI IIB criteria. Re-MI, repeat myocardial infarction; NS, not significant.

have improved the benefits of the angioplasty arm. The single factor which may affect the extension of provision of primary angioplasty facilities is that of cost comparison. Some of the studies mentioned above have involved cost comparisons and have shown similar or marginal benefits with angioplasty; however, until definitive data regarding long-term outcomes are available, such comparisons are not valid.

Stenting in AMI

In all of the previously mentioned trials, there was no usage of intracoronary stents and antithrombotic regimens involved mainly aspirin and heparin. It is also interesting to note that, in all the trials, angiographic success was reported when residual stenosis was <50%. It has been shown that the degree of residual stenosis following angioplasty correlates with restenosis rates. In the PAMI II study, the only predictors of recurrent ischaemia and infarct artery reocclusion were the presence of a post-PTCA residual stenosis of >30%, the appearance of dissection or a reduced left-ventricular ejection fraction.[45,46] That the rates of angiographic restenosis or occlusion at 6 months after primary PTCA have not routinely been documented is somewhat surprising, given the suggestion above that it is this factor which may contribute to lack of long-term benefit. But it has been investigated by several workers, who have found angiographic restenosis in 37–49% and late infarct artery reocclusion in 9–14%.[26,39,47–49] This obviously may contribute to revascularization rates.

The implantation of intracoronary stents has revolutionized the practice of interventional cardiology in stable patients,[50] but can such successes be translated into the unstable situation of AMI? Ever since the first stents were implanted in 1986, doubts have been raised about the logic of implanting a metallic object with obvious thrombotic properties in a vessel where occlusion might have dire consequences.[51,52] These concerns are even more acute in the setting of an AMI, where unstable plaques, thrombus and circulating activated platelets already exist. However, if the concerns of thrombosis are laid aside for a moment, the reasons why stent implantation in these circumstances might be useful are obvious. Stents are well known to seal dissection planes and improve most post-PTCA residual stenosis in elective stenting. In AMI this can reduce recurrent ischaemia and reocclusion, thereby reducing rates of death and reinfarction. Possibly more importantly, stents are able to produce a larger lumen than PTCA alone, and this has resulted in improved clinical angiographic outcomes in an elective setting.[53–55]

Bail-out stenting in AMI

Stents were initially used cautiously in AMI, mainly for the reasons mentioned above, and tended to be used as a 'bail-out' measure for acute or threatened closure. However, evidence supporting this approach in the form of randomized controlled trials is lacking, due no doubt to lack of ethical alternatives, given that the only other alternatives to stent placement are perfusion PTCA, conservative care or emergency CABG. In a very comprehensive review of the subject, Stone[56] identified 12 studies of 'bail-out' stenting in AMI where this was performed in at least 70% of patients and with at least 50 patients included.[57–68] These studies were very heterogeneous, with differences in enrolment and procedures, so direct comparisons between them are therefore not, strictly speaking, valid. However, the review provides a good overview of the practice of 'bail-out' stenting in a selected group (Table 9.4).

Average success rates were reported at 96%, with a rate of subacute thrombosis of 3.4%. There was 5.4% early mortality, 1.2% reinfarction rate and 7.0% need for target vessel revascularization (TVR). The data for long-term follow-up are, once again, not comprehensively reported, perhaps somewhat surprisingly, given that this is the area where stents should be expected to produce significant further benefits over PTCA alone.

Table 9.4
Combined early and late meta-analysis results of bail-out stenting.

	Early	Late
No. of patients	1150	338
Success rates (%)	96	NA
Death (%)	5.4	4.8
Repeat AMI (%)	1.2	0
Stent thrombosis (%)	3.4	NR
TVR (%)	7.0	10.8

NA, not applicable; NR, not reported; Early, up to 30 days; Late, 6–18 months (mean 8.5); TVR, target vessel revascularization.

There are seven studies with 10 patients or more reporting long-term follow-up for an average of 8.5 months,[61,63,64,67,69–71] but even these data are not complete. TVR rates at 8 months were reported as 10.8%, with a composite rate of death, reinfarction or TVR of 13.3%, data which do seem to represent a significant improvement over PTCA. The angiographic restenosis rate in a subset was found to be 26% with an 87% angiographic restudy at 6 months.

The practice of routine stent placement after an acceptable primary PTCA result is obtained cannot at this stage be supported, as it is not known if this confers any added benefits, but in a situation where there is severe recoil or flow-limiting dissection, bail-out stenting can unequivocally be recommended. The question of residual stenoses of 30–50% and non-flow-limiting dissections awaits the publication of further studies. Recommendations on post-stenting pharmacological regimens must include aspirin, ticlopidine (which will be discussed later) and, perhaps controversially, intravenous or low molecular weight heparin for at least 3 days. The use of heparin post-primary stenting has not been investigated, particularly in the current setting of widespread use of antiplatelet agents.

Primary stenting versus PTCA

The safety and feasibility of a primary stent approach where stents are implanted in all patients irrespective of angioplasty result has been evaluated by a number of non-randomized studies, although there are a growing number of randomized studies either ongoing or recently published looking at this area. A review[56] of six non-randomized studies, including 10 or more patients reporting the outcome of a primary stent strategy in AMI, has been published.[72–77] A total of 544 patients was included, with a success rate of 98%. The combined rate of subacute thrombosis was low at 1.8%, as were the short-term (<3 months) rates of death (0.9%), reinfarction (1.3%), CABG (1.8%) and repeat TVR (2.1%). The combined end-point of death, reinfarction or TVR was 6.1%. These results would seem to be a significant improvement over PTCA alone, but selection bias cannot be ruled out. The late results are not reported or are ongoing, but results would tend to suggest a restenosis rate of between 15% and 25% at 6 months.[72,76] The PAMI Stent Pilot trial

investigation, which was the largest of these trials, concluded that a primary stent strategy in AMI is safe and feasible in the majority of patients undergoing mechanical reperfusion.[72] They recommended routine high-pressure implantation techniques to ensure greater stent apposition.

Having conclusively demonstrated that a primary stent strategy is safe, the priority is now to demonstrate by randomization that it is superior to angioplasty alone in the treatment of AMI. The review identifies six randomized trials which have recently presented their results or are ongoing (Table 9.5).[56,78–81] In the Florence Randomised Elective Stenting in Acute Coronary Occlusions (FRESCO) Trial,[78] 150 patients were randomized to stenting or no further

Table 9.5
Results of randomized trials of primary stenting (quoted first) versus primary PTCA.

	FRESCO[78]	ESCOBAR[79]	PASTA[80]	STENTIM[56]	GRAMI[81]
Patient numbers	150	204	142	220	104
Crossover rate (%)	0	13	10	23.5	25
Stent success (%)	100	98	97	96	98
Mortality (%)	1 versus 0	0.5 versus 1.5	3.3 versus 8.2	4.1 versus 3.9	–
Reinfarction (%)	1 versus 3	0.5 versus 1.5	–	2.1 versus 6.1	–
TVR (%)	7 versus 25[a]	2 versus 10[b]	5 versus 13.1	2.1 versus 12.2[e]	11.5 versus 15.5
Combined end-point (%)	9 versus 28[b]	3 versus 13[c]	5 versus 21.3[d]	8.2 versus 21.6[e]	17 versus 35[c]

[a]p < 0.002; [b]p = 0.03; [c]p = 0.02; [d]p < 0.008; [e]p < 0.05.
Crossover rates, crossover from PTCA to stent; TVR, target vessel revascularization; Combined end-point, total of target vessel revascularization, reinfarction or death.
ESCOBAR, 30-day results; FRESCO, 6-month results; GRAMI, 1-year results; PASTA, incomplete in-hospital results; STENTIM 2, in-hospital results.

therapy following a successful angioplasty (restoration of TIMI III flow and residual stenosis <30%). The 30-day results showed significantly fewer recurrent ischaemic events in the stented group (3% versus 15%), resulting in a significant excess of TVR in the angioplasty group (12% versus 1%). The 6-month results also showed a significant reduction in recurrent ischaemia rates and repeat TVR. The incidence of restenosis or reocclusion was 17% in the stent group and 43% in the angioplasty group. This trial differs from the others to be mentioned, in that the initial angioplasty had to be successful before randomization.

The ESCOBAR Trial[79] randomized 204 patients to primary stenting or PTCA but there was a 15% 'crossover' to stenting in the PTCA group. The results showed significantly fewer TVR in the stented group at 30 days.

The Primary Angioplasty versus Stent Implantation in AMI (PASTA) Trial[80] enrolled 142 patients, and preliminary incomplete results show a reduced composite end-point of in-hospital death, reinfarction and TVR in the stented group. Once again, there was a 'crossover' rate of 10%. The clinical results would seem to be preserved at 9 months, as are the results of restenosis and minimum luminal diameter at repeat angiography at 3 months, although all the results are not available yet.

The Gianturco Roubin II Stent in AMI (GRAMI) Trial[81] randomized 104 patients following crossing of the lesion with a guidewire. There was a much higher 'crossover' rate of 25% of PTCA patients, a fact that may explain the failure to demonstrate differences in 1-year TVR or restenosis rates, although in the stented group there was a significant improvement in freedom from the composite rate of death, reinfarction or TVR, both in hospital and at 1 year. These latter results were primarily due to decreased death and reinfarction in patients who presented in Killip class III–IV and were stented.

The Second Stent in AMI (Stentim) Trial and the PRISAM trial[56] are not yet reported, but preliminary results appear to be giving similar results to the trials above. Since Stone's review, there has been further work comparing a strategy of primary stenting to PTCA with stent 'bail-out'.[82] Overall, 94 patients received 'bail-out' stents, and were compared to 53 primary stent patients. The results suggested significantly fewer late target vessel revascularizations (18% versus 36%) and better late event-free survival (44% versus 80%) in the primary stent group.

The trials above all have the problem of having insufficient numbers of patients to show a reduction in mortality or reinfarction with a primary stent strategy alone in AMI, but they do seem to suggest that the main disadvantages of primary PTCA, late restenosis and occlusion can be significantly improved by the insertion of a stent in the majority of cases. To determine whether this will translate into improved clinical end-points, as is being implied, needs further large-scale trials.

Antiplatelet therapy

The initial reluctance to implant stents into a thrombotic environment has already been mentioned. Initially, it was thought necessary to institute an intensive anticoagulation regimen with aspirin and heparin in the immediate post-procedure period which was continued until full anticoagulation was established with a coumadin derivative for a prolonged period, and, indeed, this did result in a significant reduction in stent thrombosis from 18% to 0.6%.[51] This apparent remarkably low level of stent thrombosis has not been achieved by other workers, and the more usually quoted rate of stent thrombosis is 1–9%. However, this regimen also led to a significant increase in haemorrhagic and vascular access site complications, with the latter varying between 10% and 30%, resulting in a substantial prolongation of hospital stay.[83] Because this was one of the major factors against stenting in general, the search was then on for alternatives with fewer complications. Attention was directed towards

antiplatelet therapy, as it was shown initially in animal models that there was a rapid deposition of platelets at the stent site.[84] In humans, markers of platelet activation, surface expression of the activated fibrinogen receptor (glycoprotein IIb/IIIa), von Willibrand factor binding and P-selectin expression peaked 2 days following stent placement and coincided with a significant drop in peripheral platelet counts. These changes were not seen with angioplasty alone.[85]

Ticlopidine

Ticlopidine was the agent to which attention was drawn. Ticlopidine blocks the adenosine diphosphate (ADP)-mediated activation of platelet glycoprotein IIb/IIIa receptors.[86] For some time it has been the only true antiplatelet agent, other than aspirin, used in interventional cardiology. The addition of ticlopidine was shown to prevent platelet activation in the above study.[85] When the combination of aspirin and ticlopidine was used post stent, stent thrombosis rates were reduced to less than 2%.[87] Large-scale studies have been performed to confirm these results. The Intracoronary Stenting and Anti-thrombotic Regimen (ISAR) trial, Stent Anticoagulation Regimen Study (STARS) and Full Anticoagulation versus Ticlopidine plus Aspirin after Stent Implantation (FANTASTIC) trials have been presented. These have all shown a significant reduction in primary end-points of death, myocardial infarction or revascularization accompanied by a reduction in haemorrhagic complications when aspirin plus ticlopidine are compared to aspirin plus anticoagulation.[66,88,89] In the ISAR trial, a subgroup had stents implanted for AMI and, as already described, the 30-day clinical event rates were significantly lower (3.3% versus 21%), the 6-month freedom from recurrent AMI was better (100% versus 90.3%) and the rate of stent occlusion was lower (1.6% versus 14.5%). However, restenosis rates were similar in both groups (26.5% versus 26.9%).[90] The only disadvantage with the use of ticlopidine is the side-effect profile, which includes minor ones of rashes and gastrointestinal upset and the more important risk of neutropenia. The latter has been severe in 0.8% of cases, but usually with prolonged (2–3 months) therapy, and is often reversible on discontinuation of therapy.[87,91] The current recommended duration of therapy is 1 month following stenting, and thus the likelihood of encountering this complication is much less. The profound benefits of ticlopidine have now made its use mandatory in modern stenting practice, but because of the concerns over its side-effects, attention has been directed towards strategies of using aspirin alone. The MUSIC trial looked at the use of intravascular ultrasound to ensure optimal stent deployment and used aspirin alone with encouraging results.[92] It is unlikely, however,

that in the more actively thrombotic environment of an AMI, this course of action would produce similar results, particularly given the routine use of high-pressure stent deployment techniques already.

Recently, a new agent of the thienopyridine class, clopidogrel, has been shown to be of similar efficacy to ticlopidine in reducing stent thrombosis in the as-yet-unpublished Clopidogrel Aspirin Stent International Co-operative Study (CLASSICS). This agent has previously been proven to have a far superior side-effect profile to ticlopidine, permitting its longer-term usage.[93] It is likely that it will supersede the use of ticlopidine following stent implantation in the near future.

Glycoprotein IIb/IIIa inhibitors

The most recent weapon in the arsenal directed against thrombotic complications in interventional cardiology comprises the group of drugs which specifically inhibit the platelet GP-IIb/IIIa receptor, of which abciximab (ReoPro) is the most widely tested (Table 9.6). Initial studies were directed towards patients judged to be at high risk of complications during intervention, namely acute or recent myocardial infarction, unstable angina or complex lesion morphology.[94] The results of the EPIC trial showed a significant reduction in the composite of death, AMI or revascularization across all subgroups when

Table 9.6
Results of the randomized use of GPIIb/IIIa inhibitors (quoted first) versus placebo in intervention cases (see text for further study details).

	Patient numbers	Death (%)	MI (%)	Urgent revascularization	Composite end-point (%)	Major bleeding (%)
EPIC (6 month)	2099	1.7 versus 1.7	5.2 versus 8.6[a]	16.5 versus 22.3[b]	8.3 versus 12.8[b]	10.6 versus 3.3[c]
EPIC (unstable) (6 month)[95]	489	1.8 versus 6.6[a]	2.4 versus 11.1[b]	18.7 versus 22	25.4 versus 35[a]	9.7 versus 4.5
EPIC (3 year)[97]	2099	6.8 versus 8.6	10.7 versus 13.6	34.1 versus 40.1[a,d]	41.1 versus 47.4[b]	–
CAPTURE (30 day)[98]	1265	1.0 versus 1.3	4.1 versus 9.0[a]	7.8 versus 10.9	11.3 versus 15.9[a]	3.8 versus 1.9[a]
EPILOG (30 day)[99]	2792	0.3 versus 0.8	3.7 versus 8.7[c]	1.6 versus 5.2[c]	5.2 versus 11.7[c]	2.0 versus 3.1
EPISTENT (30 day) STENT[100]	2399	0.3 versus 0.6	4.5 versus 9.6[a]	1.3 versus 2.1	5.3 versus 10.8[c]	1.5 versus 2.2
EPISTENT (30 day) PTCA[100]	2399	0.8 versus 0.6	5.3 versus 9.6[a]	1.9 versus 2.1	0.9 versus 10.8[b]	1.4 versus 2.2

[a] $p < 0.05$; [b] $p < 0.009$; [c] $p < 0.001$; [d] All revascularization.
Composite end-point: death, MI or revascularization.

abciximab was given as a bolus followed by a 12-h infusion, but the reductions were particularly marked in those with the syndrome of unstable angina.[95,96] These differences have also, quite surprisingly, been shown to be maintained long term, up to 3 years.[97] Similar results were obtained in the CAPTURE trial;[98] here, patients with unstable angina were randomized but the results did not appear to suggest that the benefits might be prolonged beyond a few days. The disadvantage of the regimen was a significant increase in haemorrhagic complications. This fact was addressed in the EPILOG trial,[99] where patients undergoing PTCA were randomized to placebo and standard-dose heparin, abciximab and standard-dose heparin, or abciximab and low-dose heparin. Once again, significant benefits were seen in the abciximab groups and there was a reduction in minor haemorrhagic complications in the low-dose heparin group to levels similar to those of the placebo and heparin group. In all these trials, few or no stents were implanted, but in the EPISTENT trial there was a comparison between abciximab with PTCA, abciximab with stenting, and stenting alone, in elective procedures.[100] This showed a significant reduction in the combined end-point of death, AMI or urgent revascularization at 30 days in the stent plus abciximab versus stent alone group, and also in the PTCA plus abciximab group. The conclusions to be drawn are that both PTCA and stenting with abciximab appear to be safer than stenting without abciximab.

Two further trials have looked specifically at the use of GP-IIb/IIIa inhibitors in primary PTCA, the RESORE trial (using tirofibran)[101] and the RAPPORT trial,[102] and have shown decreased rates of recurrent ischaemia and TVR after primary PTCA, but the numbers have not been large enough to draw definite conclusions. It is hoped that the answers from the Controlled Abciximab and Device Investigation to Lower Late Angioplasty Complications (CADILLAC) trial will help to settle the debate.[56] In this ongoing trial, 1720 patients with AMI will be randomized to primary PTCA with placebo, primary PTCA with abciximab, primary stenting with placebo, or primary stenting with abciximab.

Heparin-coated stents

In the PAMI Heparin Coated Stent Pilot trial,[103] a specially designed Palmaz–Schatz stent which has heparin molecules bonded onto the stent surface was deployed in 101 patients undergoing primary PTCA, and intravenous heparin was not used. The results showed an excellent safety profile with no acute cardiac end-points. Consequently, the PAMI Heparin Coated Stent Randomised Trial was carried out. In this trial, 900 patients with AMI were randomized to receive the heparin-coated stent and no peri-procedural heparin versus primary PTCA and a 60-h tapering heparin regimen. The 30-day results were presented at the American College of Cardiology meeting in Atlanta in 1998, and showed non-significant reductions in death, recurrent AMI or disabling stroke, but a significant reduction in ischaemia-driven TVR (0.6% versus 2.5%). The 6-month results have been reported at the 1998 TCT conference in Washington and are essentially the same as the results in the 30-day report. This approach, using a regimen in primary stenting which does not require heparin, is likely to further reduce vascular complications and facilitate earlier discharge.

Stenting in thrombus-containing lesions

Conventional guidelines consider the presence of intracoronary thrombus to be an absolute contraindication to stenting.[51,52] However, as discussed previously, primary stenting consistently gives a better result than PTCA alone in AMI, a situation in which it is well known that the underlying pathological substrate frequently includes thrombus.[104,105] This apparent dichotomy is often explained by using the argument that if a thrombus is visible at angiography it signifies a heavy thrombus burden which may carry a higher risk for stent implantation. In a non-randomized trial, the safety of stenting in

visible thrombus-containing lesions has been demonstrated.[106] Only 22% of their patients had an AMI, but 75% had the procedure carried out for unstable angina. Procedural success rates were similar to those mentioned previously (96%). The results show low rates of subacute thrombosis (1%), death (6%) and non-Q-wave myocardial infarction (6%), with acceptable restenosis rates (33%). Definite conclusions are difficult to draw, given the non-randomized nature of the trial, but the results would tend to suggest that patients should not be denied stenting purely on the basis of a thrombus being visible.

It is likely that the use of GP IIb/IIIa inhibitors in the setting of stent implantation in thrombus-containing lesions will further improve results, as data from the EPIC trial would suggest. Here, the presence of thrombus during angioplasty alone did predict a higher rate of subacute occlusion. However, the significant benefits of abciximab already mentioned were of the same order of magnitude whether or not thrombus was present.[107] Definitive trial work in this area is still awaited.

In conclusion, primary PTCA has been shown to give consistently better reperfusion rates than thrombolytic therapy, with better short- and long-term outcomes. These benefits are further improved by stent implantation in selected cases, which can help prevent many of the complications associated with primary PTCA alone. The optimal antithrombotic regimen includes short-term heparin which needs to be weight adjusted, especially if a GP IIb/IIIa inhibitor is to be given, and ticlopidine if a stent is to be implanted.

PTCA following thrombolysis has no place in routine AMI care, but for those with evidence of failed thrombolysis, ongoing ischaemia or contraindications to thrombolysis, further benefits can be achieved by mechanical intervention.

The cost-effectiveness of the newer and often very expensive developments has to be carefully weighed in each patient population before routine use is encouraged. For many hospitals, the option of primary mechanical treatment of AMI is not feasible and the mainstay of therapy will still be thrombolytic agents. In the majority of settings, thrombolytic therapy still provides very significant improvements in morbidity and mortality. It is difficult to envisage how a therapy with such ease and speed of administration will ever lose its place at the top of the therapeutic ladder for AMI. Indeed, for those with the facilities available, the choices are in some ways more difficult, given the necessity to provide dedicated infrastructure and personnel 24 h per day; the finance required to do this is not likely to be made available in many countries, except in a few dedicated centres.

Hopefully, this review shows the results of what can be achieved. In many enthusiasts' eyes, the Rubicon has been crossed, but for many others the complexities of offering such a service may prove insurmountable.

References

1. Goldman L, Cooke EF, The decline in ischaemic heart disease mortality rates. An analysis of the comparative effects of medical interventions and changes in lifestyle, *Ann Intern Med* 1987; **101**: 825.

2. Beaglehole R, Medical management and decline in mortality from coronary heart disease, *Br Med J* 1986; **292**: 33.

3. ISIS-2 Collaborative Group, Randomised trial of intravenous streptokinase, oral aspirin, both, or neither among 17,187 cases of suspected acute myocardial infarction, *Lancet* 1988; **ii**: 349–60.

4. Yusef S, Peto R, Lewis J, Colleris R, Sleight P, Beta blockade during and after myocardial infarction: an overview of the randomised trials, *Prog Cardiovas Dis* 1985; **27**: 335–71.

5. Simoons ML, Myocardial infarction: ACE-inhibitors for all? For ever? *Lancet* 1994; **66**: 478–82.

6. Gruppo Italiano per lo Studio della Streptochinasi nel'Infarto Miocardico (GISSI), Effectiveness of intravenous thrombolytic treatment in acute myocardial infarction, *Lancet* 1986; **1**: 397–402.

7. Granger CB, Califf RM, Topol EJ, Thrombolytic therapy for acute myocardial infarction. A review, *Drugs* 1992; **44**: 293–325.

8. The GUSTO Investigators, An international

randomised trial comparing four thrombolytic strategies for acute myocardial infarction, *N Engl J Med* 1993; **329:** 673–82.

9. The GUSTO Angiographic Investigators, The effects of tissue plasminogen activator, streptokinase, or both on coronary artery patency, ventricular function, and survival, after acute myocardial infarction, *N Engl J Med* 1993; **329:** 1615–22.

10. Hochmann JS, Choo H, Limitation of myocardial infarct expansion by reperfusion independent of myocardial salvage, *Circulation* 1987; **75:** 299–306.

11. Kennedy JW, Ritchie JL, Davis KB et al, The Western Washington randomised trial of intracoronary streptokinase in acute myocardial infarction, *N Engl J Med* 1985; **312:** 1073–8.

12. Serruys WW, Wijns W, van den Brand M et al, Is transluminal angioplasty mandatory after successful thrombolysis? *Br Heart J* 1983; **50:** 257–65.

13. Harrison DG, Ferguson DW, Collins SM et al, Rethrombosis after reperfusion with streptokinase: importance of geometry of individual lesions, *Circulation* 1984; **69:** 991–6.

14. Erbel R, Pop T, Henrichs KJ et al, Percutaneous transluminal coronary angioplasty after thrombolytic therapy: a prospective randomised controlled trial, *J Am Coll Cardiol* 1986; **8:** 485–95.

15. Serruys PW, Simoons ML, Suryapranata H et al, Preservation of global and regional left ventricular function after early thrombolysis in acute myocardial infarction, *J Am Coll Cardiol* 1986; **7:** 729–42.

16. De Bono DP, The European Co-operative Study Group Trial of intravenous recombinant tissue-type plasminogen activator and conservative therapy versus rt-PA and immediate coronary angioplasty, *J Am Coll Cardiol* 1988; **12:** 20A–3A.

17. The TIMI Research Group, Immediate vs. delayed catheterisation and angioplasty following thrombolytic therapy for acute myocardial infarction: TIMI IIA results, *JAMA* 1988; **260:** 2849–58.

18. Topol EJ, Califf RM, George BS et al, A randomised trial of immediate vs. delayed angioplasty after tissue plasminogen activator in acute myocardial infarction, *N Engl J Med* 1987; **317:** 581–8.

19. Califf RM, Topol EJ, George BS et al, Characteristics and outcome of patients in whom reperfusion with intravenous tissue type plasminogen activator fails: results of the Thrombolysis and Angioplasty in Myocardial Infarction (TAMI) I trial, *Circulation* 1988; **77:** 1090–9.

20. Abottsmith CW, Topol EJ, George BS et al, Fate of patients with acute myocardial infarction with patency of the infarct related vessel achieved with successful thrombolysis versus rescue angioplasty. *J Am Coll Cardiol* 1990; **16:** 770–8.

21. Ross AM, Lundergan CF, Rohrbeck SC et al, Rescue angioplasty after failed thrombolysis: technical and clinical outcomes in a large thrombolysis trial, *J Am Coll Cardiol* 1998; **31:** 1511–17.

22. Ellis SG, da Silva ER, Heyndricks G et al, Randomised comparison of rescue angioplasty with conservative management of patients with early failure of thrombolysis for anterior myocardial infarction, *Circulation* 1994; **90:** 2280–4.

23. The CORAMI Study Group, Outcome of attempted rescue coronary angioplasty after failed thrombolysis for acute myocardial infarction, *Am J Cardiol* 1994; **74:** 172–4.

24. Gibson CM, Cannon CP, Green RM et al, Rescue angioplasty in the Thrombolysis in Myocardial Infarction (TIMI-4) trial, *Am J Cardiol* 1997; **80:** 21–6.

25. The Global Use of Strategies to Open Occluded Coronary Arteries in Acute Coronary Syndromes (GUSTO IIb) Angiographic Substudy Investigators, *N Engl J Med* 1997; **336:** 1621–8.

26. O'Neil WW, Weintraub R, Grines CL et al, A prospective, placebo-controlled, randomised trial of intravenous streptokinase and angioplasty versus lone angioplasty therapy of acute myocardial infarction, *Circulation* 1992; **86:** 1710–17.

27. Meier B, Balloon angioplasty for acute myocardial infarction. Was it buried alive? *Circulation* 1990; **82:** 2243–5.

28. Simoons ML, Maggioni AP, Knatterud G et al, Individual risk assessment for intracranial haemorrhage during thrombolytic therapy, *Lancet* 1993; **342:** 1523–8.

29. Grines CL, Browne KF, Marco J et al, A comparison of immediate angioplasty with thrombolytic therapy for acute myocardial infarction, *N Engl J Med* 1993; **328:** 673–9.

30. Zijlstra F, de Boer MJ, Hoorntje JCA et al, A comparison of immediate coronary angioplasty with intravenous streptokinase in acute myocardial infarction, *N Engl J Med* 1993; **328:** 680–4.

31. Gibbons RJ, Holmes DR, Reeder GS et al, Immediate angioplasty compared with the administration of a thrombolytic agent followed by conservative treatment for myocardial infarction, *N Engl J Med* 1993; **328:** 685–91.

32. Zijlstra F, Beukema W, van't Hof A et al, Randomised comparison of primary coronary angioplasty with thrombolytic therapy in low risk patients with acute myocardial infarction, *J Am Coll Cardiol* 1997; **27:** 908–12.

33. Weaver WD, Simes RJ, Betriu A et al, Comparison of primary coronary angioplasty and intravenous thrombolytic therapy for acute myocardial infarction. A quantitative review, *JAMA* 1997; **278:** 2093–8.

34. Ribeiro EE, Silva LA, Carneiro R et al, Randomised trial of direct coronary angioplasty versus intravenous streptokinase in acute myocardial infarction, *J Am Coll Cardiol* 1993; **22:** 376–80.

35. Grinfeld L, Berrocal D, Belardi J et al, Fibrinolytics vs primary angioplasty in acute myocardial infarction, *J Am Coll Cardiol* 1996; **27** (suppl): A-222.

36. DeWood MA, Direct PTCA vs intravenous t-PA in acute myocardial infarction: results from a prospective randomised trial. In: *Proceedings from the Thrombolysis and Interventional Therapy in Acute Myocardial Infarction Symposium VI* (George Washington University: Washington, DC, 1990) 28–9.

37. Ribichini F, Steffenino G, Dellavalle A et al, Primary angioplasty versus thrombolysis in inferior myocardial infarction with anterior ST-segment depression: single center randomised study, *J Am Coll Cardiol* 1996; **27:** A-222.

38. Garcia E, Elizaga J, Soriano J et al, Primary angioplasty versus thrombolysis with t-PA in the anterior myocardial infarction, *J Am Coll Cardiol* 1997; **29**(suppl A): A-389.

39. Nakagawa Y, Iwasaki Y, Kimura T et al, Serial angiographic follow-up after successful direct angioplasty for acute myocardial infarction, *Am J Cardiol* 1996; **78:** 980–4.

40. Cragg DR, Freidman HZ, Bonema JD et al, Outcome of patients with acute myocardial infarction who are ineligible for thrombolytic therapy, *Ann Intern Med* 1991; **115**: 173–7.

41. O'Keefe JO, Bailey WL, Rutherford BD et al, Primary angioplasty for acute myocardial infarction in 1000 consecutive patients, *Am J Cardiol* 1993; **72**: 107G–15G.

42. Stone GW, Grines CL, Browne KF et al, Outcome of different reperfusion strategies in thrombolytic 'eligible' versus 'ineligible' patients with acute myocardial infarction, *J Am Coll Cardiol* 1995; **25**: 401A.

43. Stone GW, Grines CL, Browne KF et al, Primary angioplasty reduces recurrent ischaemic events compared to t-PA in myocardial infarction: implications for early discharge, *Circulation* 1993; **88**: I-105A.

44. Ryan TJ, Bauman WR, Kennedy JW et al, Guidelines for percutaneous transluminal coronary angioplasty: a report of the American College of Cardiology/American Heart Association task force on assessment of diagnostic and therapeutic cardiovascular procedures (committee on percutaneous transluminal coronary angioplasty), *J Am Coll Cardiol* 1993; **22**: 2033–55.

45. Grines CL, Brodie B, Griffin J et al, Which primary PTCA patients may benefit from the new technologies? *Circulation* 1995; **92**: I-146.

46. Benzuly KH, O'Neill WW, Brodie B et al, Predictors of maintained infarct artery patency after primary angioplasty in high risk patients in PAMI-2, *J Am Coll Cardiol* 1996; **27**(suppl A): 279A.

47. Rothbaum DA, Linnemeier TJ, Landin RJ et al, Emergency percutaneous transluminal coronary angioplasty in acute myocardial infarction: a 3 year experience, *J Am Coll Cardiol* 1987; **10**: 264–72.

48. Brodie BR, Grines CL, Ivanhoe R et al, Six month clinical and angiographic follow-up after direct angioplasty for acute myocardial infarction, *Circulation* 1994; **25**: 1710–17.

49. Nakae I, Fujita M, Fudo T et al, Relation between pre-existent coronary collateral circulation and the incidence of restenosis after successful coronary direct angioplasty for acute myocardial infarction, *J Am Coll Cardiol* 1996; **27**: 1688–92.

50. De Feyter P, Foley D, Coronary stenting: has the Rubicon been crossed? *Heart* 1996; **75**: 109–10.

51. Schatz RA, Baim DS, Leon M et al, Clinical experience with the Palmaz–Schatz coronary stent: initial results of a multicenter trial, *Circulation* 1991; **83**: 148–61.

52. Agrawal SK, Ho DSV, Liu MW et al, Predictors of thrombotic complications after placement of a flexible coil stent, *Am J Cardiol*, 1994; **73**: 1216–19.

53. Serruys PW, de Jaegere P, Kiemenij F et al, A comparison of balloon expandable stent implantation with balloon angioplasty in patients with coronary artery disease, *N Engl J Med* 1994; **331**: 489–95.

54. Fischman DL, Leon MB, Baim DS et al, A randomised comparison of coronary stent placement and balloon angioplasty in the treatment of coronary artery disease, *N Engl J Med* 1994; **331**: 496–501.

55. Versaci F, Gaspardone A, Tomai F et al, A comparison of coronary artery stenting with angioplasty for isolated stenosis of the proximal left anterior descending artery, *N Engl J Med* 1997; **336**: 817–22.

56. Stone GW, Stenting in acute myocardial infarction: observation studies and randomised trials, *J Invas Cardiol* 1998; **10**(suppl A):16A–26A.

57. Steffenino G, Chierchia S, Fontanelli A et al, Use of stents during emergency coronary angioplasty in patients with high risk acute myocardial infarction: in-hospital results from the Italian multicenter registry (RAI) *Eur Heart J* 1997; **18**: 272.

58. Monassier J, Elias J, Raynaud J et al, The French registry of stenting at acute myocardial infarction, *J Am Coll Cardiol* 1996; **27**: 68A.

59. Steinhubl SR, Moliterno DJ, Teirstein PS et al, Stenting for acute myocardial infarction. The early United States experience, *J Am Coll Cardiol* 1996; **27**: 279A.

60. Glatt B, Stratiev V, Guyon B et al, Two years' experience of primary stenting in unselected acute myocardial infarction: one month follow-up, *Eur Heart J* 1997; **336**: 817–22.

61. Spaulding C, Cador R, Benhamda K et al, One week and six month angiographic controls of stent implantation after occlusive and non occlusive dissection during primary balloon angioplasty for acute myocardial infarction, *Am J Cardiol* 1997; **79**: 1592–5.

62. Neuman FJ, Walterh, Richardt G et al, Coronary Palmaz–Schatz stent implantation in acute myocardial infarction, *Heart* 1996; **75**: 121–6.

63. Repetto S, Onofri M, Castiglioni B et al, Stenting of the infarct related artery during complicated acute myocardial infarction, *J Invas Cardiol* 1996; **8**: 177–83.

64. Schomig A, Neuman FJ, Kastrati A et al, A randomised comparison of antiplatelet and anticoagulant therapy after the placement of coronary artery stents, *N Engl J Med* 1996; **334**: 1084–9.

65. Levy G, de Boisgelin R, Volpilière R et al, Intracoronary stenting in direct angioplasty: is it dangerous? *Circulation* 1995; **92**: I-131.

66. Horstkott D, Piper C, Anderson D et al, Stent implantation in acute myocardial infarction: results of a pilot study with 80 consecutive patients, *Eur Heart J* 1996; **17**: 297.

67. Hans-Jurgen R, Thomas V, Jurgen T et al, Short and long term results of stent implantation within 12 hours of failed PTCA in acute myocardial infarction, *Circulation* 1996; **94**: I-577.

68. Himbert D, Juliard JM, Benamer H et al, Hospital outcomes after bail-out coronary stenting in patients with acute myocardial infarction, *Eur Heart J* 1997; **18**: 125.

69. Rodriquez AE, Fernandez M, Santaera O et al, Coronary stenting in patients undergoing percutaneous transluminal coronary angioplasty during acute myocardial infarction, *Am J Cardiol* 1996; **77**: 685–9.

70. Setiha ME, El Gamal M, Koolen J et al, Coronary stenting for failed angioplasty in acute myocardial infarction, *Cathet Cardiovasc Diagn* 1996; **39**: 149–54.

71. Ahmad T, Webb JG, Carara R, Dodek A, Coronary stenting for acute myocardial infarction, *Am J Cardiol* 1995; **76**: 77–80.

72. Stone GW, Brodie BR, Griffin JJ et al, A prospective multicenter study of the safety and feasibility of primary stenting in acute myocardial infarction: in-hospital and 30 day results of the PAMI Stent Pilot Trial, *J Am Coll Cardiol* 1998; **31**: 23–30.

73. Declan JL, Garcia E, Soriano J et al, Primary coronary stenting in acute myocardial infarction: in-hospital results, *Eur Heart J* 1997; **18**: 275.

74. Saito S, Hosokawa G, Kim K et al, Primary

stent implantation in acute myocardial infarction, *J Am Coll Cardiol* 1996; **28:** 74–81.

75. Valeix BH, Labrunie PJ, Massiani PF et al, Systemic coronary stenting in the first eight hours of acute myocardial infarction, *Circulation* 1996; **94:** I-557.

76. Medina A, Hernandez E, Suarez de Lesco J et al, Primary stent treatment for acute myocardial infarction, *Rev Esp Cardiol* 1996; **94:** I-576.

77. Turi ZG, McGinnity JG, Fischman D et al, Retrospective comparative study of primary intracoronary stenting versus balloon angioplasty for acute myocardial infarction, *Cathet Cardiovasc Diagn* 1997; **40:** 235–9.

78. Antoniucci D, Santoro GM, Bolognese L et al, A clinical trial comparing primary stenting of the infarct related artery with optimal primary angioplasty for acute myocardial infarction: results from the Florence Randomised Elective Stenting in Acute Coronary Occlusions (FRESCO) Trial, *J Am Coll Cardiol* 1998; **31:**1234–9.

79. Hoorntje JC, Suryapranata H, de Boer MJ et al, ESCOBAR: primary stenting for acute myocardial infarction: preliminary results of a randomised trial, *Circulation* 1996; **94:** I-570.

80. Saito S, Hosokawa G, Suzuki S et al, Primary stent implantation is superior to balloon angioplasty in acute myocardial infarction—the result of the Japanese PASTA (Primary Angioplasty versus Stent Implantation in Acute Myocardial Infarction) trial, *J Am Coll Cardiol* 1997; **29:** 390A.

81. Rodriguez A, Fernandez M, Bernardi V et al, Coronary stents improved hospital results during coronary angioplasty in acute myocardial infarction: preliminary results of randomised controlled study (GRAMI trial), *J Am Coll Cardiol* 1997; **29:** 221A.

82. Mahdi NA, Lopez J, Leon M et al, Comparison of primary coronary stenting to primary balloon angioplasty with stent bailout for the treatment of patients with acute myocardial infarction, *Am J Cardiol* 1998; **81:** 957–63.

83. Steinhubl SR, Lincoff AM, Antithrombotic therapy with intracoronary stenting, *Heart* 1997; **78**(suppl 2): 21–3.

84. Parsson H, Cwikiel W, Johanssen K et al, Deposition of platelets and neutrophils in porcine iliac arteries after angioplasty and Wallstent placement compared with angioplasty alone, *Cardiovasc Intervent Radiol* 1994; **17:** 190–6.

85. Gawaz M, Neumann FJ, Ott I et al, Platelet activation and coronary stent implantation. Effect of antithrombotic therapy, *Circulation* 1996; **94:** 279–85.

86. Gershlick AH, Antiplatelet therapy following stent deployment, *Heart* 1997; **78**(suppl 2): 24–6.

87. Laplanch JM, McFadden FP, Bonnet JL et al, Combined antiplatelet therapy with ticlopidine and aspirin, *Eur Heart J* 1996; **17:** 1373–80.

88. Stent Anticoagulation Regimen Study (STARS), Presented at the American Heart Association Scientific Sessions, November 1996.

89. Bertrand ME, Legrand V, Boland J et al, Randomized multicenter comparison of conventional anticoagulation versus antiplatelet therapy in unplanned and elective coronary stenting. The full anticoagulation versus ticlopidine (fantastic) study, *Circulation* 1998; **98:** 1597–603.

90. Schomig A, Neumann FJ, Walter H et al, Coronary stent placement in patients with acute myocardial infarction: comparison of clinical and angiographic outcome after randomisation to antiplatelet or anticoagulant therapy, *J Am Coll Cardiol* 1997; **29**: 28–34.

91. Colombo A, Hall P, Nakamura S et al, Intracoronary stenting without anticoagulation accomplished with intravascular guidance, *Circulation* 1995; **90**: 1676–88.

92. De Jaegere P for the MUSIC study investigators, In hospital and one month clinical results of an international study testing the concept of IVUS guided optimised stent expansion alleviating the need for systemic anticoagulation, *J Am Coll Cardiol* 1996; 27(suppl A):731–5.

93. CAPRIE steering committee, A randomized, blinded trial of clopidogrel versus aspirin in patients at risk of ischaemic events (CAPRIE), *Lancet* 1996; **348**: 1329–39.

94. The EPIC Investigators, Prevention of ischaemic complications in high risk angioplasty by a chimeric monoclonal antibody e7E3 Fab fragment directed against the platelet glycoprotein IIb/IIIa receptor, *N Engl J Med* 1994; **330**: 956–61.

95. Topol EJ, Califf RM, Weisman HF et al, Randomised trial of coronary intervention with antibody against platelet IIb/IIIa integrin for reduction of clinical restenosis: results at six months, *Lancet* 1994; **343**: 881–6.

96. Lincoff AM, Califf RM, Anderson KM et al, Evidence for the prevention of death and myocardial infarction with platelet membrane glycoprotein IIb/IIIa receptor blockade by Abcimab (c7E3 Fab) among patients with unstable angina undergoing percutaneous coronary revascularisation, *J Am Coll Cardiol* 1997; **30**: 149–56.

97. Topol EJ, Ferguson JJ, Weisman HF et al, Long term protection from myocardial events in a randomised trial of brief integrin B3 blockade with percutaneous coronary intervention, *JAMA* 1997; **278**: 479–84.

98. The CAPTURE Investigators, Randomised placebo-controlled trial of abciximab before and during coronary intervention in refractory unstable angina: the CAPTURE study, *Lancet* 1997; **349**: 1429–35.

99. The EPILOG Investigators, Platelet glycoprotein IIb/IIIa receptor blockade and low dose heparin during percutaneous coronary revascularisation, *N Engl J Med* 1997; **336**: 1689–96.

100. The EPISTENT Investigators, Randomised placebo-controlled and balloon angioplasty-controlled trial to assess safety of coronary stenting with the use of platelet glycoprotein IIb/IIIa blockade, *Lancet* 1998; **352**: 87–92.

101. The RESTORE Investigators, Effect of platelet glycoprotein IIb/IIIa blockade with tirofiban on adverse cardiac events in patients with unstable angina or acute myocardial infarction undergoing coronary angioplasty, *Circulation* 1997; 77: 1445–53.

102. Brener SJ, Barr LA, Burchenal JE et al, for the RAPPORT investigators, Randomized, placebo-controlled trial of platelet glycoprotein IIb/IIIa blockade with primary angioplasty for acute myocardial infarction, *Circulation* 1998; **98**: 734–41.

103. Grines CL, Morice MC, Mattos L et al, A prospective, multicenter trial using the JJIS heparin-coated stent for primary reperfusion of acute myocardial infarction, *J Am Coll Cardiol* 1997; **29**: 170A.

104. Davies MJ, Thomas A, Thrombosis and acute coronary lesions in sudden cardiac ischaemic death, *N Engl J Med* 1984; **310:** 1137–40.

105. Falk E, Shah PK, Fuster V, Coronary plaque disruption, *Circulation* 1995; **92:** 657–71.

106. Alfonso F, Rodriguez P, Phillips P et al, Clinical and angiographic implications of coronary stenting in thrombus containing lesions, *J Am Coll Cardiol* 1997; **29:** 725–33.

107. Kahn MM, Ellis SG, Aguirre FV, Does intracoronary thrombus influence the outcome of high risk percutaneous transluminal coronary angioplasty? Clinical and angiographic outcomes in a large multicenter trial, *J Am Coll Cardiol* 1998; **31:** 31–6.

Surgery and the management of mechanical complications of myocardial infarction

Inderpaul Birdi and Stephen R Large

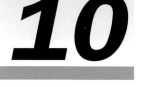

Introduction

Mechanical complications following myocardial infarction occur as a result of regional or global myocardial muscle damage. These complications include the development of myocardial and mitral valve insufficiency, malignant ventricular arrhythmias, presence of ongoing life-threatening ischaemia, ventricular septal rupture and ventricular free wall rupture, and mural clot formation and the attendant risks of systemic embolization. The late sequelae include ventricular aneurysm formation and global pump failure leading to intractable heart failure. All of these lesions have potentially serious haemodynamic consequences and are generally associated with a poor prognosis. Advances in strategies for myocardial protection, operative technique and perioperative intensive care have redefined the role of early surgical intervention in many of these conditions and have improved the dismal outlook associated with medical therapy alone. The aim of this discussion is to clarify the modern surgical approaches to the management of these lesions.

Acute mitral insufficiency

Severe postinfarction mitral insufficiency is a life threatening event that is conventionally described as resulting from papillary muscle rupture, or papillary muscle dysfunction. More recently, however, it has become apparent that postinfarction mitral insufficiency in the absence of papillary muscle rupture may be due to changes in left ventricular shape and regional function, rather than papillary muscle dysfunction.[1,2] Papillary muscle necrosis and rupture with resulting acute mitral regurgitation is a catastrophic state which usually occurs within 7 days of myocardial infarction. The culprit lesion is typically the result of isolated disease of the right coronary artery or, less commonly, the circumflex artery. The infarct suffered is often relatively small and localized.[3,4] One-third of patients have a complete disruption of the papillary muscle, resulting in flailing of both the anterior and posterior mitral leaflets, while two-thirds have rupture of one or more heads, resulting in only partial prolapse of the valve mechanism.[3] In 90% of hearts, the right coronary artery supplies the posteromedial papillary muscle, which is the most commonly damaged muscle following infarction of the posterior left ventricular wall. The diagnosis is usually obvious, and is made on the basis of sudden deterioration a few days following myocardial infarction and associated with the development of a new pansystolic murmur

without clinical evidence of a thrill (in contrast to ventricular septal rupture). Echocardiography confirms the diagnosis. Attempts at medical stabilization prior to surgery result in mortality rates as high as 90%. Emergency surgical intervention, with preoperative intra-aortic balloon pump counterpulsation at the time of diagnosis, is therefore mandatory and can achieve survival rates of 75–89%.[4]

At operation, the left atrium is often small, limiting surgical access. A transatrial incision across the right atrial wall and interatrial septum can significantly improve the exposure in these circumstances. Mitral valve repair is often not possible because of necrosis of the valve mechanism, and valve replacement with concomitant coronary artery bypass grafting is the safer option. The mitral valve ring may be friable due to infarction of adjacent ventricular muscle, and care must be taken to ensure that adequate bites of tissue are taken during suturing of the prosthesis. Occasionally, ruptured papillary muscle damage is very localized, and reimplantation can be performed. Care must be taken to ensure that the reimplantation site is in viable myocardium.

The occurrence of mitral regurgitation some time following a recent myocardial infarction with the presence of ongoing ischaemia is a more common scenario than acute mitral insufficiency. It is tempting to undertake coronary revascularization under these circumstances in the belief that this alone will result in improvement in mitral valve function. Unfortunately, unless mitral regurgitation is truly episodic, the majority of these valves will continue to leak. Even mild mitral regurgitation is an independent predictor of postinfarction mortality (Fig. 10.1), and it is generally believed that this is due to geometric abnormalities of the left ventricle.[2] Under these circumstances, repair with an annuloplasty ring and coronary artery bypass grafting may be a better

approach than coronary revascularization alone.[5,6]

Malignant ventricular arrhythmias

In the acute and subacute phase of myocardial infarction, sustained ventricular arrhythmias can be caused by a number of different mechanisms. These include abnormal impulse generation, abnormal automaticity or triggered activity caused by early or delayed after-depolarizations, or by abnormalities of impulse conduction such as re-entry

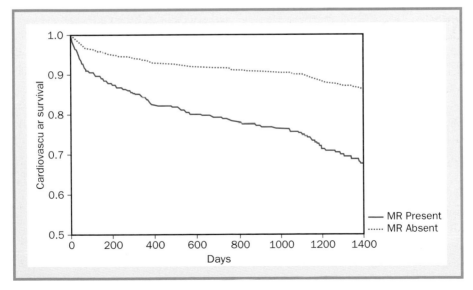

Figure 10.1
Kaplan–Meier curves of cardiovascular survival in patients with (n = 141) and without (n = 586) angiographic evidence of postinfarction mitral valve regurgitation.[2]

tachycardias.[7] These may occur within the first 48 h without necessarily affecting prognosis if treatment is prompt. If these arrhythmias occur later in the course of recovery, or are sustained, a poor long-term outcome is found even with intensive medical therapy. Depressed myocardial function is a usual finding in these patients. Radiofrequency catheter ablation therapy has become an important treatment modality for a number of tachyarrhythmias and has replaced surgical approaches in the majority of cases.[8,9] For resistant arrhythmias, the use of implantable cardioverter-defibrillators (ICD) is effective. The results of the Antiarrhythmics Versus Implantable Defibrillators (AVID) prospective randomized study have shown a mortality advantage for patients with near-fatal ventricular arrhythmias when treated with ICD insertion compared to patients receiving class III anti-arrhythmic drugs.[10] The value of ICD insertion has been confirmed in a number of other studies.[11] Implantation of ICD is relatively easy, and requires only percutaneous transvenous techniques. The device is now small enough to be placed in a subpectoral pocket.

Direct surgical ablation is a curative option for selected patients with monomorphic, sustained ventricular tachycardias, particularly in association with a ventricular aneurysm. Mapping of the myocardium is undertaken using an array of epicardial and/or endocardial electrodes. Ventricular tachycardias are induced and computer-based electrophysiological analysis is used to rapidly identify the arrhythmogenic focus. Ablation techniques can then be used to destroy these foci prior to aneurysmal surgery.

Surgical revascularization after myocardial infarction

The timing of surgical revascularization following myocardial infarction remains a controversial issue, particularly since the successful introduction of thrombolysis.[12,13] Acute haemodynamic deterioration due purely to ongoing ischaemia is a life-threatening problem that demands resuscitation with intra-aortic balloon pump support and early surgical revascularization in order to save life. The operative mortality is as high as 50%, and sophisticated techniques for myocardial preservation are generally required. It is not widely appreciated that the area often in most need of urgent revascularization may not be the region of infarction but an area remote from this region that still remains potentially salvageable.

Most surgeons also believe that the lack of resolution of ischaemia following myocardial infarction despite thrombolysis (characterized by recurrent angina or electrocardiographic changes) should prompt angiography, and revascularization by percutaneous angioplasty[14] or open surgery.[15–18] The previous use of anticoagulants or thrombolytic therapy does not represent a contraindication to surgery.

A more controversial issue arises with patients who present with uncomplicated myocardial infarction who have undergone cardiac catheterization for one reason or another, and have been found to harbour a 'critical' surgical lesion. Lee et al[19] studied 1181 consecutive patients who underwent isolated coronary revascularization between 1992 and 1995. A subgroup of 316 patients with recent myocardial infarction (less than 21 days) were subdivided into four groups according to increasing clinical severity (Table 10.1). Mortality in the non-myocardial infarction group was 2.5%. For patients with previous myocardial infarction, the death rate increased

from 1.2% in patients with stable angina, to 26% in patients in cardiogenic shock. Multivariate logistic regression identified left ventricular dysfunction, intra-aortic balloon pump pulsation and renal insufficiency as the only independent predictors of mortality. Other studies have confirmed the higher risk of surgery in patients with post-myocardial infarction unstable angina and impaired left ventricular function.[20,21]

Ventricular septal rupture

The ventricular septum receives blood from perforating branches of the left anterior descending artery, as well as perforating branches of the posterior descending artery. Despite this dual blood supply, there is frequently no septal collateral flow and, consequently, the interventricular septum

Table 10.1
Operative mortality for coronary artery bypass surgery.

Clinical severity	Number	Mortality (%)
Non-myocardial infarction	865	2.5
Post-myocardial infarction		
Stable	166	1.2
Unstable	107	3.7
IABP support	20	28.0
Cardiogenic shock	23	26.0

IABP, intra-aortic balloon pump.
Data from Lee et al.[19]

remains vulnerable to ischaemia. Myocardial infarction is complicated by rupture of the ventricular septum (VSR) in 1–2% of cases and usually occurs as a complication of a first acute myocardial infarction.[22] The anteroapical area is the most common site and is involved in 65% of patients. The posterior segment of the septum is involved in 17% of cases, and the middle segment is involved in 13%; only 4% of ruptures affect the inferior part of the septum. VSRs may be found at multiple sites and may develop, not simultaneously, but within several days of one another. Of particular note is the fact that a posterior VSR may be associated with acute mitral regurgitation.

VSR occurs 3–7 days following acute myocardial infarction. The first sign is the development of a pansystolic murmur (associated with a thrill), followed by sudden and progressive haemodynamic deterioration as the magnitude of the left-to-right shunt increases. Echocardiography confirms the diagnosis. Angiography should be performed when possible, to identify the presence and distribution of coronary arterial disease. If the patient's condition permits, the left venticulogram can be useful in identifying the site and magnitude of the VSR. Intra-aortic balloon pump counterpulsation is almost always used to improve the haemodynamic state of the patient.

Treated medically, VSR is associated with an unacceptably high mortality, approaching 25% at 24 h, 75% at 7 days, and 90% at 2 months.[23,24] The current approach, therefore, is to consider emergency surgical intervention.[24–28] The only exception to this is the rare occurrence of complete absence of haemodynamic instability that is sometimes seen with a small defect. These patients need to be carefully monitored, however, since the rupture may increase in size as continued necrosis of the septum occurs.

The surgical approach for anteriorly located VSRs is through the left ventricular infarct. It is now generally believed that debridement of infarcted tissue should be avoided as far as possible. The modern technique takes advantage of the natural pressure differential between the right and left ventricles. A 'haemodynamic patch' consisting of pericardium and dacron velour is sutured over the septum using prolene sutures placed in normal myocardium far from the infarcted septum. The object is to hold the patch on the left ventricular side of the septum and to rely upon the pressure differential to provide a blood seal. The patch is usually incorporated into closure of the ventriculotomy. With this technique, should additional septal necrosis occur, breakdown and recurrence of VSR is not an absolute certainty.

The approach to rupture of the posteroinferior aspect of the septum through the infarcted left ventricular wall is fraught with danger. Often, the posteromedial papillary muscle is involved, and concurrent mitral valve replacement may be required. When the VSR is small, the septal patch is sewn to the free wall of the right ventricle with interrupted mattress sutures to obliterate the VSR. When it is large, two patches may need to be employed, one to close the VSR, and the other to close the left ventricle. If the apex of the heart is infarcted, it is amputated. The viable tissue is then reapproximated in a sandwich fashion by means of four teflon

strips, using a series of horizontal mattress sutures. It should be remembered that concomitant coronary revascularization should be undertaken in all cases.

Only 32% of patients who survive surgical intervention are alive at 10 years (Fig. 10.2). This is related in part to the high surgical mortality (20–50%) and the poor residual ventricular function in these patients because of extensive myocardial scarring. Preoperative shock,[22,29,30] posterior site of infarction,[22,27,29] short interval between infarction and VSR

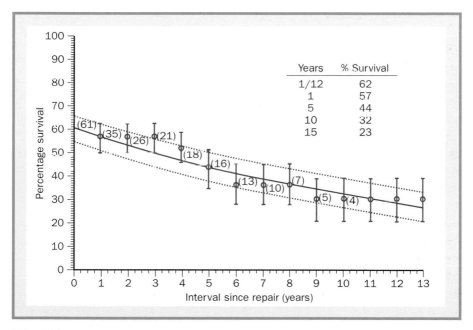

Figure 10.2
Survival after repair of postinfarction ventricular septal rupture.[26]

occurrence[29] and impaired right ventricular function due to infarction are specifically associated with poor surgical survival.[22,27,31]

Residual VSR has been noted early or late postoperatively in 10–25% of patients.[29] This may be due to reopening of a closed defect, presence of an overlooked defect, or the development of a new defect. Reoperation is generally advised when the pulmonary–systemic bloodflow ratio is greater than 2.0. This should be delayed only if the patient is haemodynamically stable with no evidence of heart failure or pulmonary hypertension.

Ventricular free wall rupture and pseudoaneurysm formation

Ventricular free wall rupture complicates approximately 4% of myocardial infarctions and accounts for 12–21% of deaths after infarction.[32] It is of note that this incidence is higher than for isolated rupture of the ventricular septum or isolated papillary muscle rupture.

Survival following free wall rupture is extremely rare. In this entity, blood leaks into the necrosing muscle fibres of the left ventricular free wall and escapes under pressure into the pericardium. This usually occurs 1 week following infarction. If pericardial adhesions are not present at this stage, cardiac tamponade and death occurs rapidly. The most common site of rupture is the anterior[33] or lateral wall.[34] There is some evidence to suggest that thrombolysis may marginally reduce the incidence of cardiac rupture (1.7% in 533 patients having thrombolysis versus 2.7% in 807 patients without treatment) following myocardial infarction.[35]

The onset of rupture may be associated with severe chest pain that is not relieved by opiates, and, ultimately, the classical features of cardiac tamponade will become apparent. The finding of electromechanical dissociation should prompt attempts at periocardiocentesis. There is usually no time for coronary angiography, and immediate surgical intervention is the only option to prevent death. The aim of surgery is to relieve tamponade and repair of the ventricular rupture. Classically, this is undertaken by infarctectomy and replacement with a prosthetic patch using cardiopulmonary bypass.[36,37] A more conservative approach is now favoured by some centres. Simple mattress suture buttressed with teflon,[38] or application of a patch to the epicardial surface with biological glue,[39] have been used with good results. When the defect is on the anterior or lateral surface of the heart, simple repair without cardiopulmonary bypass can be achieved.[39] As circumstances rarely permit preoperative coronary angiography, it is reasonable to perform life-saving surgery and plan later angiography and coronary revascularization, Alternatively, some authors suggest empirical coronary revascularization at the time of cardiac repair to minimize the risks of repeated infarction.[40]

Should cardiac rupture occur subsequent to the first week following infarction, or in a patient with pericardial adhesions, there is a possibility that blood loss can be contained, with the subsequent development of a pseudoaneurysm. The diagnosis of this extremely rare event is usually made weeks to months following myocardial infarction. Patients may be asymptomatic, or manifest symptoms secondary to coronary artery disease or as a result of the mass effect from an enlarging pseudoaneurysm. Echocardiography delineates the lesion vividly. A pseudoaneurysm is at very high risk of rupture and should be operated upon at the time of diagnosis. The pseudoaneurysm is often very thin and friable, and manipulation should be avoided prior to institution of cardiopulmonary bypass to prevent rupture. Communication with the ventricular cavity is usually via a small opening into the flase sac, which should be identified and closed using a buttressed haemoshield graft.[41]

True ventricular aneurysm formation

In contrast to pseudoaneurysms, a true ventricular aneurysm is a well-delineated transmural fibrous scar that is virtually devoid of cardiac muscle and exhibits a paradoxical movement during the cardiac cycle. In over half of patients, the endocardial surface is lined with mural thrombus. The wall of the aneurysm may calcify, making excision and ventricular reconstruction difficult. Left ventricular aneurysm (LVA) formation is thought to complicate 4–20% of patients suffering transmural myocardial infarction.[42] About 85% of LVAs are located anterolaterally near the apex. Only 5–10% of aneurysms are located on the posterior, or inferior, surface of the heart, and nearly 50% of these are actually false aneurysms. True posterior wall aneurysms are associated with a high incidence of postinfarction mitral regurgitation secondary to papillary muscle damage. The prognosis of patients with LVA is known to be poor, with an estimated 5-year mortality as high as 88% using medical therapy alone.[42]

The classic indications for surgery are the presence of associated complications which include congestive cardiac failure, embolization of intracavity thrombus, angina and ventricular arrhythmia. Surgery is performed with cardiopulmonary bypass and left ventricular venting via the right superior pulmonary vein, or main pulmonary artery. It is wise to avoid mobilization of the aneurysm prior to cross-clamping the aorta, in order to prevent systemic embolization of intramural thrombus. However, some authors have performed LVA surgery on a beating heart without aortic cross-clamping, with no adverse effects.[42] This is often necessary when performing endocardial mapping procedures in patients with LVA-associated arrhythmias. The aneurysm is resected and the left ventricle repaired using either a linear or patch technique. Resection and linear repair is performed first by opening the belly of the aneurysm widely from its basal and apical limits. Scarred, non-contractile tissue is then removed, leaving a rim of fibrous tissue for approximation. Direct endocardial excision can also be performed if indicated by epicardial or endocardial mapping. Closure of the aneurysm is then undertaken using a linear technique between teflon strips. The alternative patch technique, termed ventricular endoaneurysmorraphy, was first described by Cooley.[43] In this technique, the ventriculotomy is performed through an incision 2 cm lateral and parallel to the left anterior descending artery for anterior aneurysms, or through the aneurysm when found posteriorly. The transition between normal and scarred myocardium is found and the extent of the defect in the ventricular wall is then assessed. An oval patch of pericardium

or dacron can then be used to patch the area, using sutures secured to the intracavity rim. A portion of the lateral wall may be excised. After decalcification of the rim of the aneurysm, the ventriculotomy is then repaired using a continuous double row of sutures, care being taken to avoid damaging the left anterior descending artery. The operation is completed with coronary artery bypass grafting as appropriate. Cooley claims a number of benefits of patch repair over linear approximation. The patch technique obviates the need for long strips of teflon, with their attendant risk of infection. It may also better preserve the geometry of the left ventricle, and spares the left anterior descending artery, which can then be revascularized to improve septal blood supply. This technique can also be used to repair calcified aneurysms.[44] Finally, the aneurysmal portion of the interventricular septum can be excluded from the 'new' ventricular cavity using the patch repair. Kesler et al have compared the linear and patch techniques and have found no significant differences in mortality, angina, congestive heart failure, or echocardiographic variables.[45] Komeda et al also detected no differences in mortality among the different repair techniques, except in patients with a low ejection fraction, in whom improved survival was seen with non-linear closure.[46] Functional and anatomical outcome as assessed by echocardiography and magnetic resonance imaging are significantly improved with both linear and patch repair.[42]

The mortality of surgery falls between 2% and 18%, and surgery is successful in improving symptoms and quality of life (Fig. 10.3). Severe, non-aneurysmal left ventricular wall motion abnormalities and major arrhythmia have both been identified as factors that increase operative risk.[47] It is now known that aneurysm formation has drastic effects, not only in the infarct zone, but also on remote, viable, contractile muscle. Increased diameter of the left ventricle leads to increased wall tension, further depressing myocardial function. Some authors now believe that patients with sizeable aneurysms should be followed by serial echocardiography and nuclear imaging. Any progressive increase in

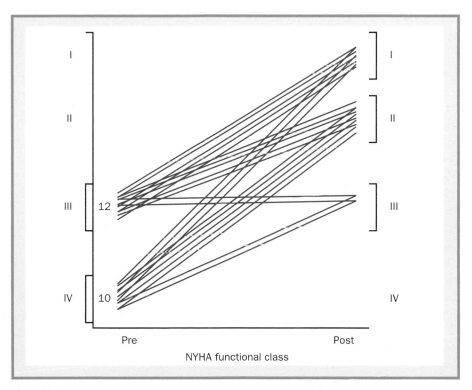

Figure 10.3
New York Heart Association functional class 1 year after patch aneurysmectomy repair presurgery and postsurgery.[64]

size of aneurysm or depression of ejection fraction may justify surgical correction.[42] This will require further study.

Surgery for heart failure

A long-term consequence of myocardial infarction is congestive heart failure. A number of surgical options are available for the treatment of this end-stage disease, and they will now be discussed briefly.

Approximately 40–50% of patients with advanced heart failure who are considered for cardiac transplantation have coronary artery disease as their underlying cause. These patients have a combination of completely infarcted and ischaemic myocardium and, with medical therapy alone, have a poor prognosis.[48] A number of cardiac imaging techniques can provide evidence of myocardial viability in these patients. These include positron emission tomography, nuclear stress imaging, dobutamine stress echocardiography, and magnetic resonance imaging. No large trials have yet evaluated the ability of viability testing to predict the clinical benefit of revascularization. Therefore, the decision to revascularize these patients is a clinical one based upon the surgeon's perceived ability to revascularize an area of potentially viable myocardium. Coronary revascularization in this population can be undertaken successfully in up to 40% of patients initially referred for

transplantation,[48] with excellent survival.[49] If revascularization is not possible, then patients should be listed for cardiac transplantation.

Orthotopic cardiac transplantation is no longer regarded as an experimental procedure, but a definitive therapeutic option for selected patients with advanced heart failure, with good long-term survival (Fig. 10.4). The decision of whether a patient will do well with medical therapy or transplantation has become a moving target as both new medical therapies and improved immunosuppressive protocols have been developed. It is envisaged that the number of patients placed onto cardiac transplant waiting lists will continue to outstrip the supply of donor organs.[50] The potential for xenotransplantation has been reduced by concerns over transmission of retroviruses from animal donors to the human pool. There is also a subset of individuals who may not be candidates for transplantation because of an expected poor outcome. These factors have fuelled the search for other surgical therapies for advanced heart failure.

Cardiomyoplasty was first described by Carpentier et al, and involves wrapping the failing dilated ventricle with a latissimus dorsi muscle flap. The neurovascular bundle is preserved and the muscle wrap is performed via a lateral thoracotomy and median sternotomy.[51] Pacing wires are appropriately placed and connected to a myostimulator

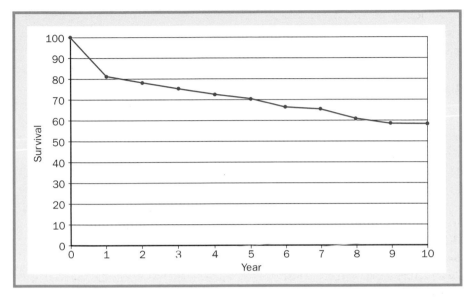

Figure 10.4
Actuarial survival following primary heart transplantation at Papworth Hospital from 1988 to 1998.

implanted in the upper chest to allow conditioning of the muscle flap at a time following surgery when the muscle flap has adhered to the epicardial surface of the left ventricle. This usually takes 2–3 weeks. Chronic, graded, low-frequency electrical stimulation is then applied to the muscle wrap to transform its behaviour from a fast, type II fatigueable muscle, to a slow, fatigue-resistant type I muscle. In the two largest series published, initial survival in patients in New York Heart Association (NYHA) class IV was very poor.[52,53] This may be due to the time delay between major surgery and possible

clinical benefit while conditioning of the muscle wrap is achieved. In addition, improvements in haemodynamics are at best modest, and inconsistent. Conversely, patients in NYHA class III seem to show some symptomatic benefit, although, again, haemodynamic measurements show inconsistent improvement. Pathological evaluation of the chronically stimulated muscle flap has demonstrated fatty degeneration of muscle with fibrous tissue replacement.[54] In addition, the risk of sudden death from arrhythmias in this population is high, and myostimulators with pacemaker and defibrillation characteristics are under development. Thus, several limitations of cardiomyoplasty have yet to be addressed before this surgical modality can be used successfully in patients with advanced heart failure.

In 1996, Batista et al reported data on more than 400 patients with dilated cardiomyopathy and described partial resection of the left ventricular muscle mass with (extrapapillary) or without (intrapapillary) mitral valve replacement.[55] Despite the lack of systematic data to demonstrate its efficacy, attempts are being made to evaluate this operation in a number of centres in Europe and North America.[56,57] The New Technology Assessment Committee for the Society of Thoracic Surgeons has suggested 'a consensus conference for the purposes of unifying protocols, patient selection and data base management'.[58] Ultimately, the value of left ventricular volume reduction surgery as a bridge to transplantation, or for the surgical treatment of patients who are not suitable for transplantation (compared to medical treatment), can only be determined in the context of a carefully controlled, randomized trial.

Transmyocardial laser revascularization (TMLR) is an investigational procedure that is being used in patients with refractory ischaemia not amenable to revascularization. The rationale of the procedure is based upon the observation that a carbon dioxide laser could create myocardial channels from the epicardium to the left ventricular cavity that are evident on gross and microscopic evaluation.[59] The effects of TMLR are far from clear, since many published reports have lacked proper controls, or have subjected patients to concomitant procedures such as coronary revascularization. Symptomatic improvement has been demonstrated by some workers following TMLR.[60,61] However, TMLR has not been shown to improve ventricular function, and although the occurrence of neoangiogenesis has been demonstrated in a pig model,[62] it has yet to be shown in humans. Results from randomized studies comparing patients who are treated medically with those who undergo TMLR will be helpful in establishing the benefits and limitations of this procedure,[63] and are currently awaited.

Finally, mechanical assist devices have been studied and used for several decades in patients with cardiogenic shock. Devices were initially developed for cardiac support after acute myocardial infarction or to assist weaning of a stunned myocardium from cardiopulmonary bypass. Continued development has allowed expansion of the use of these devices for prolonged bridging to cardiac transplantation and, more recently, as a possible alternative to cardiac transplantation. Long-term issues regarding the use of a mechanical device for permanent assistance include risks of thromboembolism, infection and device durability. Presently, heart transplantation, with its attendant limitations of donor shortage and requirements for immunosuppression, is the only effective long-term treatment for patients with advanced heart failure.

Summary

Advances in myocardial preservation and operative techniques during cardiac surgery have improved the previously dismal outlook for patients who develop acute mechanical complications following myocardial infarction. A low index of clinical suspicion will allow early diagnosis. Rapid referral for surgical intervention will require a clear understanding between cardiologists and cardiothoracic surgeons regarding the benefits and limitations of surgery in these patients. A number of surgical modalities are under investigation for patients with end-stage heart failure resistant to medical therapy that may offer some hope to patients considered unsuitable for cardiac transplantation.

References

1. Van Dantzig JM, Delemarre BJ, Koster RW et al, Pathogenesis of mitral regurgitation in acute myocardial infarction: importance of changes in left ventricular shape and regional function, *Am Heart J* 1996; **131**: 865–71.

2. Lamas GA, Mitchell GF, Flaker GC et al, Clinical significance of mitral regurgitation after acute myocardial infarction, *Circulation* 1997; **96**(3): 827–33.

3. Barbour DJ, Roberts WC, Rupture of left ventricular papillary muscle during acute myocardial infarction. Analysis of 22 necropsy cases, *J Am Coll Cardiol* 1996; **8**: 138–53.

4. Rankin JS, Hickey MJ, Smith LR et al, Ischaemic mitral regurgitation, *Circulation* 1989; **79**(suppl I): I:116–21.

5. Dion R, Ischaemic mitral regurgitation: when and how should it be corrected? *J Heart Valve Dis* 1993; **5**: 536.

6. David TE, Techniques and results of mitral valve repair for ischaemic mitral regurgitation, *J Cardiovasc Surg (Torino)* 1994; **9**(suppl 2): 274.

7. Ducceschi V, Di Micco G, Sarubbi B et al, Ionic mechanisms of ischaemia related ventricular arrythmias, *Clin Cardiol* 1996; **19**(4): 325–31.

8. Stevenson WG, Ellison KE, Lefroy DC et al, Ablation therapy for cardiac arrhythmias, *Am J Cardiol* 1997; **80**(8A): 56G–66G.

9. Rothman SA, Hsia HH, Cossu SF et al, Radiofrequency catheter ablation of post-infarction ventricular tachycardia: long term success and the significance of inducible nonclinical arrhythmias, *Circulation* 1997; **96**(10): 3499–508.

10. The AVID Investigators, A comparison of

antiarrhythmic drug therapy with implantable defibrillators in patients treated from near fatal ventricular arrhythmias, *N Engl J Med* 1997; **337:** 1576–83.

11. JP Causer, Connelly DT, Implantable defibrillators for life threatening ventricular arrhythmias, *Br Med J* 1998; **317:** 762–3.

12. ISIS-2 (Second International Study of Infarct Survival) Collaborative Group, Randomised trial of intravenous streptokinase, oral aspirin, both, or neither among 17,187 cases of suspected acute myocardial infarction, *Lancet* 1988; **2:** 349–60.

13. Rogers WJ, Baim DS, Gore JM et al, Comparison of immediate invasive, delayed invasive, and conservative strategies after tissue-type plasminogen activator. Results of the Thrombolysis in Myocardial Infarction (TIMI) Phase II-A Trial, *Circulation* 1990; **81:** 1457.

14. O'Keefe JH, Bailey WL, Rutherford BD, Hantzler GO, Primary angioplasty for acute myocardial infarction in 1000 consecutive patients. Results in an unselected population and high-risk subgroups. *Am J Cardiol* 1993; **72:** 107G–15G.

15. Kouchoukas NT, Murphy S, Philpott T et al, Coronary artery bypass grafting for postinfarction angina pectoris, *Circulation* 1989; 79(suppl I): I-68.

16. Gardner TJ, Stuart RS, Greene PS et al, The risk of coronary bypass surgery for patients with postinfarction angina, *Circulation* 1989; 7(suppl I): I-79.

17. Wasvary H, Shannon F, Bassett J et al, Timing of coronary artery bypass grafting after acute myocardial infarction, *Am Surg* 1977; 63(8): 710–15.

18. Sergeant P, Blackstone E, Meyns B, Early and late outcome after CABG in patients with

evolving myocardial infarction, *Eur J Cardiothorac Surg* 1997; **12:** 1–19.

19. Lee J, Murrell H, Strony J et al, Risk analysis of coronary bypass surgery after acute myocardial infarction, *Surgery* 1997; **122:** 675–81.

20. Jones R, Pifarre R, Sullivan H et al, Early myocardial revascularisation for postinfarction angina, *Ann Thorac Surg* 1987; **44:** 159–63.

21. Fremes S, Goldman B, Weisel R et al, Recent preoperative myocardial infarction increases the risk of surgery for unstable angina, *J Cardiovasc Surg* 1991; **6:** 2–12.

22. Moore CA, Nygaard TW, Kaiser DL et al, Postinfarction ventricular septal rupture: the importance of location of infarction and right ventricular function in determining survival, *Circulation* 1986; 74: 45–5.

23. Cooley D, Belmonte B, Zeis L et al, Surgical repair of ruptured ventricular septum following acute myocardial infarction, *Surgery* 1957; **41:** 930–7.

24. Dagget W, Buckley M, Atkins C et al, Improved results of surgical management of post-infarction septal defect, *Ann Thorac Surg* 1982; **196:** 269–77.

25. Heitmiller R, Jacobs ML, Daggett WM, Surgical management of postinfarction ventricular septal rupture, *Ann Thorac Surg* 1986; **41:** 683–91.

26. Deville C, Fontan F, Chevalier JM et al, Surgery of postinfarction ventricular septal defect: risk factors for hospital death and long term results, *Eur J Cardiothorac Surg* 1991; **5:** 167–75.

27. Jones MT, Schofield PM, Dark JF et al, Surgical repair of acquired ventricular septal defect: determinants of early and late

outcome, *J Thorac Cardiovasc Surg* 1987; **93:** 680–6.

28. Norell MS, Gershlick AH, Pillai R et al, Ventricular septal rupture complicating myocardial infarction: is earlier surgery justified? *Eur Heart J* 1987; **8:** 1281–6.

29. Skillington PD, Davies RH, Luff AJ et al, Surgical treatment for infarct-related ventricular septal defects. Improved early results combined with analysis of late functional status, *J Thorac Cardiovasc Surg* 1990; **99:** 798–808.

30. Loisance DY, Lordez JM, Deleuze PH et al, Acute post-infarction septal rupture: long term results, *Ann Thorac Surg* 1991; **52:** 474–8.

31. David TE, Dale L, Sun Z, Postinfarction ventricular septal rupture: repair by endocardial patch with infarct exclusion, *J Thorac Cardiovasc Surg* 1995; **110:** 1315–22.

32. Pohjola-Sentonen S, Muller JE, Stone PH et al, Ventricular septal and free wall rupture complicating acute myocardial infarction: experience in the multicentre investigation of limit action of infarct size, *Am Heart J* 1989; **117:** 809–18.

33. Batts KP, Ackermann DM, Edwards WD, Postinfarction rupture of the left ventricular free wall: clinicopathologic correlates in 100 consecutive autopsy cases, *Hum Pathol* 1990; **21:** 530–5.

34. Bates RJ, Beutler S, Resnekov L et al, Cardiac rupture—challenge in diagnosis and management, *Am J Cardiol* 1977; **40:** 429–37.

35. Nakamura F, Minamino T, Higashino Y et al, Cardiac free wall rupture in acute myocardial infarction: ameliorative effect of coronary reperfusion, *Clin Cardiol* 1992; **15:** 244–50.

36. Kirklin JW, Barratt-Boyes BG, eds, *Cardiac Surgery* (Churchill Livingstone, 1993) 398.

37. Yamazaki T, Eguchi S, Miyamura H et al, Replacement of myocardium with Dacron prosthesis for complication of acute myocardial infarction, *J Cardiovasc Surg (Torino)* 1989; **30:** 277–30.

38. Chemnitus JM, Schmidt T, Wojcik J et al, Successful surgical management of left ventricular free wall rupture in the course of myocardial infarction, *Eur J Cardiothorac Surg* 1991; **5:** 51–5.

39. Oliva PB, Hammill SC, Edwards WD, Cardiac rupture, a clinically predictable complication of acute myocardial infarction: report of 70 cases with clinicopathologic correlations, *J Am Coll Cardiol* 1993; **22:** 720–6.

40. Sutherland FW, Guell FJ, Pathi VL et al, Postinfarction ventricular free wall rupture: strategies for diagnosis and treatment, *Ann Thorac Surg* 1996; **61:** 1281–5.

41. Khonsari S, *Cardiac Surgery: Safeguards and Pitfalls in Operative Technique* (Lippincott-Raven, 1997) 167–8.

42. Elefteriades JA, Solomon I.W, Mickleborough LL et al, Left ventricular aneurysmectomy in advanced left ventricular dysfunction, *Cardiol Clin* 1995; **13**(1): 59–72.

43. Cooley DA, Ventricular endoaneurysmorrhaphy: results of an improved method of repair, *Texas Heart Inst J* 1989; **16:** 72–89.

44. Cooley DA, Repair of the calcified ventricular aneurysm, *Ann Thorac Surg* 1990; **49:** 489–90.

45. Kesler KA, Fiore AC, Naunhein KS et al, Anterior wall left ventricular aneurysm repair, a comparison of linear versus circular closure. *J Thorac Cardiovasc Surg* 1992; **103:** 841–8.

46. Komeda M, Cavid TE, Malik A et al,

Operative risks and long term results of operation for left ventricular aneurysm, *Ann Thorac Surg* 1992; **53**: 22–9.

47. Cohen M, Packer M, Gorlin R, Indications for left ventricular aneurysmectomy, *Circulation* 1983; **67**: 717–22.

48. DiCarli MF, Davidson M, Little R et al, Value of metabolic imaging with positron emission tomography for evaluating prognosis in patients with coronary artery disease and left ventricular dysfunction, *Am J Cardiol* 1994; **73**: 527–33.

49. Elefteriades JA, Tolis G Jr, Levi E et al, Coronary artery bypass grafting in severe left ventricular dysfunction: excellent survival with improved ejection fraction and functional state, *J Am Coll Cardiol* 1993; **22**: 1411–17.

50. The US Scientific Registry for Transplant Recipients and The Organ Procurement and Transplantation Network, *UNOS 1996 Annual Report* (USSRTRTOPTN 1996): 1–410.

51. Carpentier A, Chachques JC, Acar C et al, Dynamic cardiomyoplasty at seven years, *J Thorac Cardiovasc Surg* 1993; **106**: 42–54.

52. Moriera LFP, Stolf NAG, Bocchi EA et al, Clinical and left ventricular function outcomes up to five years after dynamic cardiomyoplasty, *J Thorac Cardiovasc Surg* 1995; **109**: 353–63.

53. Furnary AP, Jessup M, Moriera LFP, Multicentre trial of dynamic cardiomyoplasty for chronic heart failure, *J Am Coll Cardiol* 1996; **28**: 1175–80.

54. Kalil-Filho R, Bocchi E, Weiss RG et al, Magnetic resonance imaging evaluation of the chronic changes in latissimus dorsi cardiomyoplasty, *Circulation* 1995; **90**: 102–6.

55. Batista RJV, Santos JLV, Takehita N et al, Partial left ventriculotomy to improve left ventricular function in end stage heart disease, *J Cardiovasc Surg* 1996; **11**: 96–7.

56. Birdi I, Bryan AJ, Mehta D et al, Left ventricular volume reduction surgery, *Int J Cardiol* 1997; **62**(suppl 1): S29–35.

57. Starling RC, Young JB, Scalia GM et al, Preliminary observations with ventricular remodelling for refractory congestive heart failure, *J Am Coll Cardiol* 1997; **29**: 64.

58. New Technology Assessment Committee, Left ventricular reduction. *Ann Thorac Surg* 1997; **63**: 909–10.

59. Kohmoto T, Fisher PE, Gu A et al, Physiology, histology and 2 week morphology of acute transmyocardial channels made with a carbon dioxide lase, *Ann Thorac Surg* 1997; **63**: 1275–83.

60. Frazier OH, Cooley DA, Kadipasaoglu KA et al, Myocardial revascularisation with laser. Preliminary findings, *Circulation* 1995; **92**(suppl 2): 58–65.

61. Horvath KA, Mannting F, Cummings N et al, Transmyocardial laser revascularisation: operative techniques and clinical results at two years, *J Thorac Cardiovasc Surg* 1996; **111**: 1047–53.

62. Mueller X, Tevaearai H, Genton C et al, Transmyocardial laser revascularisation in acutely ischaemic myocardium, *Eur J Cardiothorac Surg* 1998; **13**: 170–5.

63. Wallwork J, Schofield P, Caine N et al, Health technology assessment: TMR trials and tribulations, *Lancet* 1996; **348**: 1386.

64. Donato M, Sabatier M, Montiglio F et al, Outcome of left ventricular aneurysmectomy with patch repair in patients with severely depressed pump function, *Am J Cardiol* 1995; **76**: 557–61.

Arrhythmias associated with acute myocardial infarction

Rana A Sayeed and Andrew A Grace

Introduction

Cardiac arrhythmias are almost universal in patients with acute myocardial infarction (AMI) and range from the benign and clinically insignificant to the frankly life-threatening. Most of the deaths in the first hour after coronary occlusion are well recognized as being due to ventricular arrhythmias.[1,2] Large datasets have now been obtained from the controlled clinical trials of thrombolysis documenting the prevalence and assigning some significance to arrhythmias occurring in patients with AMI.[3,5] When these are applied together with previous observational data, a consensus view appears to emerge as to how to manage arrhythmias around the time of myocardial infarction and before discharge from hospital. These approaches are not entirely evidence-based, but mortality from arrhythmias during periods of monitoring on coronary care units is now low, and further significant reductions in arrhythmic deaths in this period seem unlikely. There remain, however, many questions regarding the reduction of arrhythmia risk in patients following hospital discharge.

Ventricular arrhythmias

Mechanisms of ventricular arrhythmias

Ventricular arrhythmias are common in AMI.[6] Ischaemia is a metabolic insult functionally defined by the loss of normal cardiac mechanical and electrical activity, and the effects of myocardial ischaemia on normal cardiac electrophysiology have been extensively reviewed.[7] The infarct zone is the usual source of arrhythmias and is an evolving heterogeneous mass of tissue. The disturbance of conduction of the cardiac impulse is unevenly distributed, and this provides the substrate for ventricular arrhythmias, most usually due to re-entry.[7] For the development of ventricular arrhythmias, another factor, such as a premature ventricular beat or change in heart rate, must act as a trigger on the substrate (Fig. 11.1). The outcome of this interaction between trigger and substrate is influenced by many factors which modulate arrhythmogenic risk. Factors tending to enhance such risk include electrolyte imbalance (hypokalaemia, hypomagnesaemia), metabolic derangement (hypoxia, acidosis), continuing ischaemia (occluded infarct-related artery), and sympathetic overactivity (both locally released and circulating catecholamines, the latter elevated by pain or anxiety).

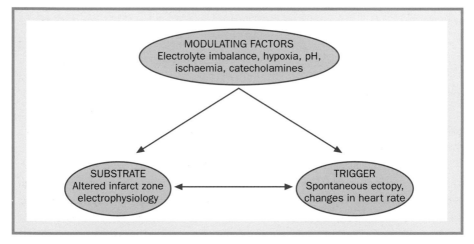

Figure 11.1
The interaction between substrate, triggers, and modulating factors in the initiation of ventricular arrhythmias after acute myocardial infarction.

Reperfusion arrhythmias

The restoration of flow down the infarct-related artery may result in the appearance of reperfusion arrhythmias including ventricular premature beats (VPBs), accelerated idioventricular rhythm, non-sustained ventricular tachycardia (NSVT) and ventricular fibrillation (VF).[1,8] Such arrhythmias are, of course, non-specific but have been suggested to reflect successful reperfusion.[8] Although there is apparently a higher incidence of reperfusion arrhythmias following severe ischaemia of short duration, a meta-analysis of trials documenting the success of thrombolysis showed no increase in the risk of VT or VF in patients receiving thrombolysis compared to those receiving placebo.[9] Accordingly, the use of prophylactic anti-arrhythmic therapy to cover thrombolysis is not recommended.

Ventricular premature beats

VPBs are common in AMI, being observed in more than 90% of patients,[1,2,6] with ~20% of patients having frequent (>10 per hour) VPBs.[6] It has generally been assumed that VPBs could trigger malignant ventricular arrhythmias, particularly when exhibiting multiform morphology, repetitive patterns such as couplets or triplets, or early coupling (the R-on-T phenomenon). In view of these concerns, the routine administration of lignocaine (lidocaine) prophylaxis to suppress these VPBs and thus reduce the risk of VT or VF became popular.[10,11] However, it was later observed that the incidence of VPBs in patients developing VF was similar to that in patients without this complication, and that only 41% of cases of VF are triggered by early-coupled VPBs.[12] In addition, overviews of trials using prophylactic lignocaine in AMI have generally found an excess of deaths in lignocaine-treated patients due to bradycardia and asystole, despite a significant reduction in the rate of primary VF.[10] Accordingly, with the low specificity of VPBs for predicting malignant ventricular arrhythmias and the lack of a mortality benefit with intravenous lignocaine, its routine use can no longer be recommended in the early phase of AMI.[11]

VPBs in the early phase of AMI are to be expected, being non-specific markers of cardiac electrical instability. Patients should be monitored to allow the early detection of malignant arrhythmias, and any potentiating factors should be sought and corrected. In particular, electrolyte imbalance (hypokalaemia and hypomagnesaemia) and persistent ischaemia must be considered. VPBs rarely produce haemodynamic compromise, but if they are frequent enough to produce hypotension, despite attention to the factors above, lignocaine can be a useful drug given as a 100-mg intravenous bolus (5 ml of 2% solution) over 30 s, followed by a maintenance infusion if required (Table 11.1).

Table 11.1
Drugs commonly used in the management of arrhythmias associated with myocardial infarction

Drug	Indication	Dose	Side-effects
Lignocaine	(Frequent VPBs) VT Refractory VF	Bolus: 100 mg (1.0–1.5 mg/kg) IV, then 50–100 mg if needed up to a total of 200 mg (3 mg/kg) Infusion: 4 mg/min for 30 min, then 2 mg/min for 2 h, then 1 mg/min for 6–24 h	Drowsiness, confusion, parasthesiae, seizures
Amiodarone	VT Refractory VF AF	Loading: 300 mg (5 mg/kg) IV over 1 h, then 900 mg (15 mg/kg) IV over 23 h, and/or 200 mg tds PO for 7 days, then 200 mg bd for 7 days Maintenance: 200 mg od	Photosensitivity, skin pigmentation, thyroid dysfunction, pulmonary fibrosis
Magnesium	VT AF	10 mmol Mg^2 IV (5 ml 50% magnesium sulphate)	Hypotension, flushing
Atropine	Symptomatic bradycardia (sinus bradycardia, type I Second-degree AV block) Asystole	0.5–1 mg IV, repeated up to 3 mg	Blurred vision, dry mouth, nausea, constipation, urinary retention
Adenosine	Broad-complex tachycardia Narrow-complex tachycardia AF/atrial flutter	3 mg IV, then 6 mg, then 12 mg at 2 min intervals if required	Transient chest pain, dyspnoea, flushing, nausea
Digoxin	AF	Loading: 0.5–1 mg IV in two equal doses at 0 and 4 h Maintenance: 62.5–250 µg od (according to age and renal function)	Nausea, anorexia, confusion, atrial tachyarrhythmias, junctional tachyarrhythmias, ventricular ectopics
Atenolol	AF	2.5–5 mg IV repeated up to 10 mg	Hypotension, bradycardia
Metoprolol	(Sinus tachycardia)	2.5–5 mg IV repeated up to 15 mg	
Verapamil	AF/atrial flutter Atrial tachycardia	5–10 mg IV repeated after 20 min up to a total of 20 mg	Hypotension

AF, atrial fibrillation; AV, atrioventricular block; VF, ventricular fibrillation; VT, ventricular tachycardia.

Ventricular tachycardia

Significant ventricular arrhythmias are seen in over 10% of patients with AMI[5] (Fig. 11.2). The haemodynamic consequences of VT are related to several factors, including the tachycardia cycle length and ventricular function. The main differential diagnosis of a broad-complex tachycardia is supraventricular tachycardia with aberrant conduction, well covered in other texts, but in the context of recent AMI, VT should always be considered more likely.

Accelerated idioventricular rhythm

Slow VT is often referred to as accelerated idioventricular rhythm and represents an infranodal rhythm with a rate of 50–120 beats/min.[2] It is common in the first 48 h after AMI and may also be associated with reperfusion. It is believed to arise from abnormal automaticity of ischaemic Purkinje fibres in the infarct zone. Episodes are usually transient and well tolerated, and no adverse effects on prognosis are suggested. Increasing the sinus rate with atropine or atrial pacing will generally control the ventricular rhythm if indicated to correct haemodynamic compromise.

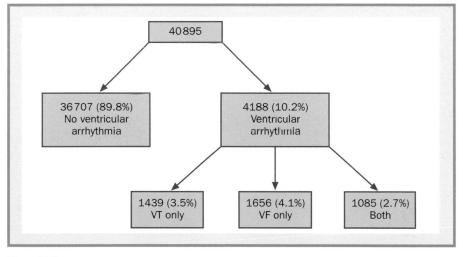

Figure 11.2
Incidence of ventricular arrhythmias in GUSTO-1. Data were available for 40 895 patients. Of these, 4188 had ventricular tachycardia (VT) only, ventricular fibrillation (VF) only, or both. Eight patients had missing data on either VT or VF. Overall, 2529 patients (6.2%) had VT and 2744 (6.7%) VF. (Adapted with permission from Circulation *1998;* **98***: 2567–73.)*

Ventricular tachycardia

Altered automaticity and increased catecholamine sensitivity in surviving subendocardial Purkinje fibres are believed to be responsible for VT arising in the first few hours. VT is defined as more than three consecutive ventricular ectopic beats with a rate greater than 120 beats/min. VT may be sustained, with episodes longer than 30 s or causing haemodynamic compromise, or non-sustained. The morphology may be monomorphic or polymorphic.

NSVT occurs in 1–7% of patients with

AMI.[13,14] The data available until recently regarding the prognosis of NSVT were limited but suggested no adverse effects on mortality.[14] The idea therefore arose that the appearance of NSVT had a significance more akin to that of VPBs than to that of sustained monomorphic VT. Recent evidence now suggests that NSVT in the setting of AMI may have a more important prognostic significance. A relatively benign outcome is expected if it occurs in the first several hours; conversely, if NSVT first appears after 8–12 h have elapsed, it is associated with increased risk[15] (Fig. 11.3). These

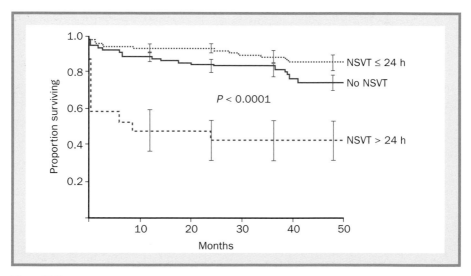

Figure 11.3
*Kaplan–Meier survival curves for AMI patients without non-sustained VT (NSVT), with NSVT within 24 h of presentation, and with NSVT after 24 h. Patients with NSVT after 24 h from presentation had poorer survival (P <0.0001) than the other two groups. (Reproduced with permission from Circulation 1998; **98**: 2030–6.)*

findings have strengthened the view that the 48-h cut-off for determining the significance of ventricular arrhythmias may need reconsideration.[15]

Polymorphic VT is uncommon, affecting ~0.3–2% of patients,[14] and is usually a marker of ongoing myocardial ischaemia best treated by anti-ischaemic interventions. Sustained monomorphic VT occurs in 0.3–1.9% of patients within 48 h of AMI[14] and is usually a sign of extensive myocardial damage and an independent marker of mortality;[16] occurring in the first 48 h, it carries a 20% in-hospital mortality, higher than other types of VT,[13] but after discharge, the survival at 1 year may be no different from that of patients with NSVT or no VT.[14] Late VT arising after the first 24 h is usually observed in extensive transmural AMI with significant left ventricular dysfunction. There are greater haemodynamic effects and this arrhythmia carries a correspondingly higher long-term mortality. Sustained VT occurring after the first day merits consideration of further investigation.

VT is detrimental because it can increase myocardial oxygen demand and opens the risk of deterioration to VF. Prompt treatment is therefore imperative but the priorities depend upon the degree of haemodynamic compromise. Rapid polymorphic or 'pulseless' VT, usually with a rate in excess of 150 beats/min, is treated as a cardiac arrest as described for VF, with a precordial thump, if appropriate, followed by an unsynchronized 200-J DC shock.[17] With lesser degrees of haemodynamic compromise seen with monomorphic VT at rates greater than 150 beats/min accompanied by angina, pulmonary congestion and hypotension, synchronized DC cardioversion is appropriate, starting with a 100-J shock.

For well-tolerated VT, often at rates less than 150 beats/min, potentiating factors such as electrolyte imbalance, hypoxia or severe acidosis should be identified and treatment initiated at the same time as anti-arrhythmic therapy. The plasma potassium concentration should be maintained at 4.5–5.0 mmol/l, and magnesium supplements should be considered, particularly if there is associated hypokalaemia, a history of diuretic therapy, or impaired left ventricular function. First-line drug treatment is with intravenous lignocaine given as a 100-mg bolus (1.0–1.5 mg/kg), which may terminate an episode of VT. Subsequent boluses of 50 mg (0.5–0.75 mg/kg) may be given every 5 min if required up to a maximum of 200 mg (3 mg/kg) loading dose (Table 11.1). A maintenance infusion should be started and continued for 6–24 h. The initial rate of 4 mg/min is halved to 2 mg/min after 30 min, and halved again to 1 mg/min after a further 2 h, to avoid toxicity. Infusion protocols should be less aggressive in old age, cardiac failure, or hepatic dysfunction. Amiodarone is an alternative and is usually used if lignocaine has proven ineffective when given according to this standard regimen. Intra-aortic balloon counterpulsation can be useful in patients with recurrent VT associated with severe ongoing post-infarct ischaemia, as a bridge to revascularization. Programmed ventricular stimulation may also occasionally be useful in the management of recurrent bouts of sustained VT. Burst pacing at 10–20 beats/min faster than the ventricular rate can terminate VTs, but carries the risk of precipitating VF.

Ventricular fibrillation

VF has a characteristic appearance and is almost uniformly lethal without prompt treatment. The incidence of VF in AMI is approximately 0.5–4%, and appears to be declining with the advent of thrombolytic therapies and the routine administration of beta-blockers, which have been shown to reduce the incidence of primary VF.[11] VF may be subdivided into three groups with different prognostic implications. Primary VF arises suddenly in the early phase of AMI, apparently as a consequence of electrical instability in the infarct zone. Sixty per cent of cases occur within 4 h and 80% within 12 h, of the onset of symptoms.[18] Secondary VF develops later in the setting of progressive

ventricular dysfunction and cardiogenic shock and is often a terminal event. Late VF that arises more than 48 h after the onset of symptoms is associated with large infarcts and significant ventricular dysfunction.

Although resuscitated primary VF increases in-hospital mortality, the long-term effects on mortality are controversial.[5] Secondary VF occurs as a function of infarct size and the extent of ventricular dysfunction and has a high in-hospital mortality. Late VF carries a poor prognosis, but this may now be open to modification with the advent of effective implantable devices (see below).

Treatment of ventricular fibrillation
VF abolishes cardiac output, and prompt defibrillation is essential. Updated guidelines for the treatment of VF and 'pulseless' VT have recently been published by the European Resuscitation Council[17] (Fig. 11.4). Suspected VF must be confirmed by rapid clinical assessment to avoid confusion caused by movement artifact or lead disconnection. Once VF has been confirmed, an unsynchronized DC defibrillating shock is given without delay and this may be repeated twice if unsuccessful. The rhythm should be reassessed after each shock and the pulse checked if the rhythm has changed to one compatible with a cardiac output. The sequence of energies of the first three shocks is: 200 J, 200 J, 360 J. Subsequent shocks are

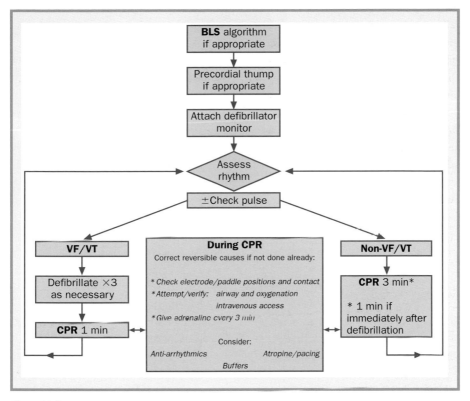

Figure 11.4
*Algorithm for adult advanced life support. CPR, cardiopulmonary resuscitation. (Reproduced with permission from Br Med J 1998; **316**: 1863–9.)*

delivered at 360 J if required. Over 80% of patients who will be successfully defibrillated respond to one of the first three shocks, but if VF persists, then cardiopulmonary resuscitation should commence. The airway must be secured, preferably by endotracheal intubation, and ventilation with 100% oxygen given. Intravenous access must be established and effective cardiac massage commenced. Adrenaline is given 1 mg intravenously or 2–3 mg via the endotracheal tube; this dose is repeated after every 3 min. After 1 min of cardiopulmonary resuscitation, another series of three shocks is given. If VF persists, the cycle is repeated. Anti-arrhythmic drugs such as lignocaine or amiodarone may be considered after three or four sets of shocks. Treatable predisposing factors such as electrolyte imbalance should be sought during resuscitation, and the administration of buffers to correct the inevitable acidosis accompanying a prolonged VF arrest should be guided by arterial blood gas analysis.

Atrial arrhythmias

Sinus bradycardia

Sinus bradycardia is a common arrhythmia usually seen with inferior or posterior AMI.[1] It is observed in up to 40% of patients within the first hour after the onset of symptoms, but the incidence declines to 15–20% after 4 h.[2] It may reflect vagal overactivity due to stimulation of cardiac vagal afferent nerve fibres, severe pain or morphine administration. It is usually a benign rhythm, needing observation only; however, heart rates less than 50 beats/min may compromise myocardial function, producing hypotension and worsening myocardial ischaemia, or may allow the development of ventricular escape rhythms.

The presence of hypotension, ischaemia or frequent VPBs indicates the need for treatment of sinus bradycardia. Intravenous atropine is used initially in doses of

0.5–1.0 mg, repeated if needed every 5 min to a total dose of 3 mg, which is usually effective in restoring the heart rate and improving hypotension or abolishing VPBs. If bradycardia is resistant to atropine, then pacing is indicated; transvenous right ventricular pacing is usually used, but in patients with marked ventricular dysfunction, dependent on the atrial contribution to cardiac output, atrial or atrioventricular (AV) sequential pacing is preferred.

Sinus tachycardia

Sinus tachycardia is observed in almost 30% of cases of AMI.[2] It is usually an appropriate physiological response to sympathetic overactivity due to ongoing chest pain, anxiety, left ventricular failure or pericarditis, but may have detrimental effects by increasing myocardial oxygen demand and reducing coronary perfusion. Management is directed at determination of the cause and appropriate treatment, for example analgesia for pain, diuretics for heart failure, or nonsteroidal anti-inflammatory drugs for pericarditis.

Atrial tachyarrhythmias

Atrial fibrillation (AF) is the commonest atrial tachyarrhythmia after AMI, with an incidence of approximately 7–18%.[3] The incidence of AF after AMI remains common, even with the increased use of thrombolysis.[3] It is usually transient, most often appearing in the first 72 h, but with only 3% arising in the early phase within 3 h of the onset of chest pain. Left atrial ischaemia is thought to be the cause of early AF, usually observed in inferior AMI secondary to occlusive disease in both the AV nodal branch of the right coronary artery and the proximal left circumflex artery before the origin of the left atrial artery.[3]

AF develops more often in older patients and those with three-vessel coronary artery disease, large infarcts, especially anterior, and poor left ventricular function.[3] Significant left ventricular dysfunction is the most important factor in AF following anterior AMI, but the occurrence of AF is also associated with pericarditis, electrolyte abnormalities such as hypokalaemia and hypomagncsaemia, and sympathetic overactivity. AF is an independent predictor of in-hospital stroke, mainly ischaemic, and 30-day mortality.[3] The incidence of systemic embolization is higher in patients with paroxysmal AF than in those without.[5]

AF is detrimental because of the increased ventricular rate and the loss of the atrial contribution to ventricular filling in the poorly compliant ischaemic ventricle. AF producing haemodynamic compromise or exacerbating myocardial ischaemia warrants synchronized DC cardioversion, with a starting energy of 100 J, then 200 J, and then 360 J if lower energies fail. In the absence of haemodynamic compromise, control of the ventricular rate may be achieved with digoxin, beta-blockers, or verapamil. Intravenous digoxin (8–15 µg/kg) given in two doses 4 h apart may produce satisfactory slowing of the ventricular rate, but the onset of action is slower than that of beta-blockade. Intravenous atenolol (2.5–5.0 mg, repeated if needed to a total of 10 mg in 10–15 min) or metoprolol (2.5–5.0 mg, repeated if needed to a total of 15 mg in 10–15 min) are effective at rapid slowing of the ventricular response, but are contraindicated in the presence of clinical left ventricular dysfunction, severe pulmonary disease, severe peripheral vascular disease, or AV block, and careful monitoring must be maintained in case of sudden falls in heart rate or blood pressure. Intravenous verapamil (5–10 mg, repeated at 15–20 min if required) is an alternative if beta-blockers are contraindicated, but it has a more marked negative inotropic effect. Heparin should be given to cover the risk of systemic embolization. Persistent AF may be treated with agents such as amiodarone, with the aim of achieving pharmacological cardioversion, and improving the success of delayed elective cardioversion if AF persists. AF associated with AMI rarely persists for more than 6 weeks, and so only a limited duration of therapy is needed. Oral anticoagulation should also be given.

Atrial flutter is rare in AMI. It is less

responsive to pharmacological agents, but is usually effectively terminated by low-energy DC cardioversion at 25–50 J or atrial overdrive pacing. Atrial tachycardia is observed in less than 10% of cases of AMI.[1] The rapid ventricular rate has the same detrimental effects on myocardial function and viability as AF. Significant hypotension demands synchronized DC cardioversion. Vagotonic manoeuvres such as carotid sinus massage or the Valsalva manoeuvre may be successful in the stable patient; otherwise, agents acting on the AV node are usually effective, such as adenosine, verapamil, or beta-blockers. Atrial overdrive pacing may be useful for recurrent atrial tachycardia.

Disturbances of cardiac conduction

The incidence and patterns of conduction disturbances in the thrombolytic era have recently been reviewed.[4] AV block of some degree develops in 12–14% of patients with AMI.[4,19,20] Early AV block, probably the result of increased vagal tone, develops within 6 h of the onset of symptoms, usually resolves within 24 h, and is responsive to atropine, with pacing rarely indicated. Late AV block develops after 6 h, is longer lasting, and is less responsive to atropine and more likely to require temporary pacing. This form of AV block is the consequence of ischaemic damage to the AV node and infranodal tissues.

Prolonged AV block is a predictor of increased in-hospital mortality, reflecting more extensive underlying myocardial damage.

First-degree AV block

First-degree AV block is observed in 4–14% of cases of AMI, usually due to intranodal conduction delay, with narrow QRS complexes. However, it is more common in anterior AMI or in association with bifascicular block, where it signifies infranodal damage and there is a higher risk of progression to complete AV block. Otherwise, first-degree AV block carries no adverse prognosis, and no specific treatment is required other than monitoring in case of progression to higher degrees of heart block.

Second-degree AV block

Mobitz type I second-degree AV block (Wenckebach) is usually a transient phenomenon, lasting less than 72 h, seen in 4–10% of cases of AMI, particularly in the inferior territory due to right coronary occlusion.[4] There is incremental intranodal delay and the QRS complex is narrow. Treatment with atropine or temporary pacing is only required if the bradycardia is poorly tolerated. The risk of progression to complete AV block is low.

Mobitz type II second-degree AV block is rare

in AMI, and when it does occur is usually seen in anterior infarction. It is the result of infranodal ischaemic damage, and the QRS complexes are wide. There is a high risk of sudden progression to complete AV block, and temporary pacing is therefore indicated.

Complete AV heart block

Complete AV block is seen in approximately 6% of cases of AMI and is more common in inferior or posterior infarction (~10.5%).[4,19,21] It carries an increased in hospital mortality related to the site and extent of infarction (anterior worse than inferior) and to the resulting damage to the AV node and infranodal conducting tissue (infranodal worse than intranodal). There has been no apparent fall in the incidence of complete AV block with the introduction of thrombolysis.[4]

Complete AV block in association with inferior infarction is usually the result of right coronary artery occlusion (the AV nodal artery is a branch of the right coronary artery in 90% of patients) producing intranodal damage and often develops gradually from lower degrees of AV block. The rhythm is usually junctional with narrow QRS complexes, and the rate greater than 40 beats/min. This form of complete AV block usually resolves over the first 1 or 2 weeks, and truly persistent complete AV block is rare.[4]

Complete AV block developing in anterior infarction often arises suddenly, on the background of bundle branch block, bifascicular or trifascicular block or Mobitz type II second-degree AV block.[4] There is extensive septal necrosis and infranodal damage; hence the escape rhythm is usually slower than 40 beats/min, with broad complexes. There is a significant risk of asystole. The prognosis is poor and is dependent on infarct size rather than the AV block. Temporary pacing is indicated for either type of complete AV block, to prevent hypotension, ischaemia and ventricular ectopy, although some cases of early narrow-complex (intranodal) complete AV block may respond to intravenous atropine alone.

Intraventricular conduction disturbances

Bundle branch block is observed in 10–20% of cases of AMI but may represent antecedent disease in up to half of the patients.[4] Right bundle branch block (RBBB) is seen in 2% of patients with AMI, usually anteroseptal with left anterior descending artery occlusion. The presence of RBBB carries a higher in-hospital and long-term morbidity and mortality, particularly in association with left ventricular dysfunction,[4,22] and it frequently progresses to complete AV block.

Left anterior hemiblock (LAHB) is identified

by left axis deviation on the ECG. It occurs in 3–5% of cases of AMI, with only a slight increase in mortality. The risk of death is higher if LAHB coexists with RBBB, signifying more extensive septal damage than in isolated LAHB. Isolated LAHB is unlikely to progress to AV block. Left posterior hemiblock (LPHB) produces right axis deviation on the ECG. It is a rare sign, observed in only 1–2% of patients with AMI.

The risk of progression from trifascicular to complete AV block is greater than 30%, and temporary pacing is indicated. The mortality is increased due to extensive myocardial damage and poor left ventricular function.

Pacing in acute myocardial infarction

Temporary pacing may be achieved using transcutaneous or transvenous approaches. External transcutaneous pacing has the advantages of being quicker to apply and non-invasive, but it is uncomfortable and not universally available. Transvenous pacing requires skilled insertion under radiographic screening and carries a risk of serious complications, including precipitation of ventricular arrhythmias, right ventricular perforation, and infection. Nonetheless, it is recommended in cases where prolonged pacing is likely or the risk of progression to complete AV block is perceived as being high.

Temporary pacing may also alleviate the haemodynamic compromise and risks of myocardial ischaemia or escape ventricular arrhythmia associated with a slow heart rate.

Permanent pacemaker implantation is rarely needed after AMI. Indications for permanent pacing are related to the degree of AV block rather than the presence of symptoms. Permanent pacing is indicated in persistent complete or Mobitz type II second-degree AV block, intermittent high-degree block in association with bundle branch block, and, very rarely, sinoatrial disease.

Reducing sudden cardiac death after hospital discharge

Risk stratification in the early phase following acute myocardial infarction

Death from myocardial infarction occurs not only during the acute phase but also later during convalescence after hospital discharge, with many deaths unheralded and presumed to be due to ventricular arrhythmias. The most important clinical markers of high risk of presumed arrhythmic death are frequent VPBs and left ventricular dysfunction;[23] there is a correlation between the frequency and repetitiveness of VPBs and increased mortality, with additive effects from reduced left ventricular ejection fraction (LVEF). Thus patients with NSVT and LVEF ≤ 0.30

following AMI have a 2-year mortality of 30%.[23] Several non-invasive measures have been tested in an attempt to identify patients at risk of sudden cardiac death. Although these can be predictive of an increased risk, their positive predictive accuracy is too low for routine screening purposes; combinations of different techniques, however, are more reliable and may prove to be of clinical use.[24]

Programmed ventricular stimulation is a commonly used method for the assessment of risk in patients with ventricular arrhythmias late after myocardial infarction. This technique is invasive and impractical, and, indeed, of limited value for screening of patients after AMI.[25]

Management of the patient at high risk of sudden cardiac death

Drug therapy
Beta-blockers have a beneficial effect on mortality and are now widely prescribed after AMI,[26,27] but there is no evidence to support the routine use of specific anti-arrhythmic therapy after AMI. Indeed, overviews of trials of prophylactic anti-arrythmic drug therapy in AMI have concluded that the routine use of class I agents was associated with increased mortality.[26] However, those patients at higher risk of ventricular arrhythmias may benefit from other appropriately targeted therapies.

There has been considerable recent interest in using class III agents in selected patients post-AMI. An early meta-analysis of several small trials found that amiodarone improved survival,[26] and two more recent, larger trials with amiodarone have also been encouraging. The European Myocardial Infarct Amiodarone Trial (EMIAT[28]) assessed the efficacy of amiodarone in post-infarct patients with reduced left ventricular function (LVEF ≤ 0.40). There was a reduction in death classified as having an arrhythmic origin but no effect on cardiac or all-cause mortality. The Canadian Amiodarone Myocardial Infarction Trial (CAMIAT[29]) used amiodarone in post-infarct patients with frequent VPBs or an episode of VT. In this study, amiodarone reduced the composite outcome of resuscitated VF and arrhythmic death, but there was no effect on total mortality. However, neither study had sufficient power to detect modest reductions in all-cause mortality. In both EMIAT and CAMIAT, concomitant beta-blockade conferred additional benefit. A more recent meta-analysis of 13 amiodarone trials that included high-risk post-AMI patients showed significant reductions in overall mortality.[30] The definitive effects of amiodarone on overall mortality remain to be shown in a large, suitably powered, prospective, randomized controlled study.

Other class III agents have also been evaluated

in randomized, controlled trials. The SWORD (Survival with oral *d*-sotalol) trial was designed to examine the effect of *d*-sotalol, a 'pure' class III agent, on all-cause mortality in survivors of AMI with left ventricular dysfunction (LVEF ≤ 0.40).[31] The study was terminated early because *d*-sotalol administration was associated with excess mortality, possibly due to pro-arrhythmic effects, particularly in the group with remote AMI and the best left ventricular function and therefore at lowest risk of ventricular arrhythmia. The results of the trials with dofetilide (DIAMOND)[32] and azimilide (ALIVE)[33] in high-risk post-infarct patients are awaited. Preliminary results from DIAMOND-MI suggest a reduction in AF arrhythmic deaths but a neutral effect on overall mortality.

Indications for the ICD
Recent trials have evaluated implantable cardioverter-defibrillators (ICDs) in high-risk patients after AMI. The Multicentre Automatic Defibrillator Implantation Trial (MADIT[34]) compared ICD therapy and anti-arrhythmic drugs for a group of 196 high-risk patients after Q-wave myocardial infarction; entry criteria included LVEF ≤ 0.35, a history of non-sustained VT and inducible sustained VT or VF not suppressed by procainamide on electrophysiological study. There was a 57% reduction in cardiac mortality over 27 months in the ICD group.[34] However, the inability of

procainamide to suppress VT predicts the failure of other anti-arrhythmic drugs, and 11% of the drug-treated group were on class I agents, which have been shown to increase mortality in this group.[26] Therapy in the drug-treated patients was therefore likely to be ineffective or possibly harmful, which may explain the large benefit seen in the ICD group. MADIT-2 and the Defibrillator in Acute Myocardial Infarction trial (DINAMIT) are currently recruiting with similar entry criteria (early post-MI, low ejection fraction and other markers of risk for arrhythmic events) and will examine the role of prophylactic ICD therapy post-MI.[35]

General approach to the reduction of long-term arrhythmia risk
On the basis of current evidence, patients with preserved left ventricular function and a low frequency of VPBs are at low risk of sudden cardiac death. Beta-blockers are routinely prescribed in the absence of any contraindications but no anti-arrhythmic agents have been shown to be of benefit in this low-risk group.[27] Patients with significant left ventricular dysfunction (LVEF ≤ 0.40) and frequent VPBs or non-sustained VT may benefit from amiodarone.

Patients with sustained VT or VF occurring beyond 24 h after AMI may merit invasive electrophysiological investigation. Therapeutic options will then include anti-arrhythmic drugs guided either by non-invasive strategies or by electrophysiological studies, or else the use of empirical amiodarone. ICDs will generally be reserved for those with recurrent ventricular arrhythmias or persistent inducibility despite anti-arrhythmic therapy who also have no significant comorbidity. Interventional approaches that include radiofrequency ablation, revascularization with percutaneous transluminal coronary angioplasty or surgery, and map-guided ventricular surgery, may all be indicated in specific patient groups. For example, patients with a defined arrhythmogenic focus, usually related to myocardial scar tissue and aneurysm formation, and/or persistent occlusive coronary artery disease, giving rise to myocardial ischaemia, may be good candidates for surgery.

References

1. Camm AJ, Redwood SR, Peri-infarction arrhythmias. In: Podrid PJ, Kowey PR, eds, *Cardiac Arrhythmia: Mechanisms, Diagnosis and Management*, 1st edn (Williams and Wilkins: Baltimore, 1995) 1239–52.

2. Antman EM, Braunwald E, Acute myocardial infarction. In: Braunwald E, ed., *Heart Disease*, 5th edn (WB Saunders: Philadelphia, 1997) 1184–288.

3. Crenshaw BS, Ward SR, Granger CB et al, Atrial fibrillation in the setting of acute myocardial infarction: the GUSTO-I experience. Global Utilization of Streptokinase and TPA for Occluded Coronary Arteries, *J Am Coll Cardiol* 1997; **30**(2): 406–13.

4. Simons GR, Sgarbossa E, Wagner G et al, Atrioventricular and intraventricular conduction disorders in acute myocardial infarction: a reappraisal in the thrombolytic era, *Pacing Clin Electrophysiol* 1998; **21**(12): 2651–63.

5. Newby KH, Thompson T, Stebbins A et al, Sustained ventricular arrhythmias in patients receiving thrombolytic therapy: incidence and outcomes. The GUSTO Investigators, *Circulation* 1998; **98**(23): 2567–73.

6. Maggioni AP, Zuanetti G, Franzosi MG et al, Prevalence and prognostic significance of ventricular arrhythmias after acute myocardial infarction in the fibrinolytic era. GISSI-2 results, *Circulation* 1993; **87**(2): 312–22.

7. Janse MJ, Wit AL, Electrophysiological mechanisms of ventricular arrhythmias resulting from myocardial ischemia and infarction, *Physiol Rev* 1989; **69**(4): 1049–169.

8. Krumholz HM, Goldberger AL, Reperfusion arrhythmias after thrombolysis. Electrophysiologic tempest, or much ado about nothing, *Chest* 1991; **99**(4 suppl): 135S–40S.

9. Solomon SD, Ridker PM, Antman EM, Ventricular arrhythmias in trials of thrombolytic therapy for acute myocardial infarction. A meta-analysis, *Circulation* 1993; **88**(6): 2575–81.

10. MacMahon S, Collins R, Peto R et al, Effects of prophylactic lidocaine in suspected acute myocardial infarction. An overview of results from the randomized, controlled trials, *JAMA* 1988; **260**(13): 1910–16.

11. Antman EM, Berlin JA, Declining incidence of ventricular fibrillation in myocardial infarction. Implications for the prophylactic use of lidocaine, *Circulation* 1992; **86**(3): 764–73.

12. El-Sherif N, Myerburg RJ, Scherlag BJ et al, Electrocardiographic antecedents of primary ventricular fibrillation. Value of the R-on-T phenomenon in myocardial infarction, *Br Heart J* 1976; **38**(4): 415–22.

13. Campbell RW, Murray A, Julian DG, Ventricular arrhythmias in first 12 hours of acute myocardial infarction. Natural history study, *Br Heart J* 1981; **46**(4): 351–7.

14. Eldar M, Sievner Z, Goldbourt U et al, Primary ventricular tachycardia in acute myocardial infarction: clinical characteristics and mortality. The SPRINT Study Group, *Ann Intern Med* 1992; **117**(1): 31–6.

15. Cheema AN, Sheu K, Parker M et al, Nonsustained ventricular tachycardia in the setting of acute myocardial infarction: tachycardia characteristics and their prognostic implications, *Circulation* 1998; **98**(19): 2030–6.

16. Mont L, Cinca J, Blanch P et al, Predisposing factors and prognostic value of sustained monomorphic ventricular tachycardia in the early phase of acute myocardial infarction, *J Am Coll Cardiol* 1996; **28**(7): 1670–6.

17. Advanced Life Support Working Group of the European Resuscitation Council, The 1998 European Resuscitation Council guidelines for adult advanced life support, *Br Med J* 1998; **316**(7148): 1863–9.

18. Volpi A, Cavalli A, Franzosi MG et al, One-year prognosis of primary ventricular fibrillation complicating acute myocardial infarction. The GISSI (Gruppo Italiano per lo Studio della Streptochinasi nell'Infarto miocardico) investigators, *Am J Cardiol* 1989; **63**(17): 1174–8.

19. Berger PB, Ruocco NA Jr, Ryan TJ et al, Incidence and prognostic implications of heart block complicating inferior myocardial infarction treated with thrombolytic therapy: results from TIMI II, *J Am Coll Cardiol* 1992; **20**(3): 533–40.

20. Nicod P, Gilpin E, Dittrich H et al, Long-term outcome in patients with inferior myocardial infarction and complete atrioventricular block, *J Am Coll Cardiol* 1988; **12**(3): 589–94.

21. Goldberg RJ, Zevallos JC, Yarzebski J et al, Prognosis of acute myocardial infarction complicated by complete heart block (the Worcester Heart Attack Study), *Am J Cardiol* 1992; **69**(14): 1135–41.

22. Ricou F, Nicod P, Gilpin E et al, Influence of right bundle branch block on short- and long-term survival after acute anterior myocardial infarction, *J Am Coll Cardiol* 1991; **17**(4): 858–63.

23. Bigger JT Jr, Fleiss JL, Kleiger R et al, The relationships among ventricular arrhythmias, left ventricular dysfunction, and mortality in the 2 years after myocardial infarction, *Circulation* 1984; **69**(2): 250–8.

24. Copie X, Hnatkova K, Staunton A et al, Predictive power of increased heart rate versus depressed left ventricular ejection fraction and heart rate variability for risk stratification after myocardial infarction. Results of a two-year follow-up study, *J Am Coll Cardiol* 1996; **27**(2): 270–6.

25. DeBelder MA, Camm AJ, Use of electrophysiological studies in patients after acute myocardial infarction, *J Cardiovasc Electrophysiol* 1991; **2**: 53–64.

26. Teo KK, Yusuf S, Furberg CD, Effects of prophylactic antiarrhythmic drug therapy in acute myocardial infarction. An overview of results from randomized controlled trials, *JAMA* 1993; **270**(13): 1589–95.

27. Freemantle N, Cleland J, Young P et al, β Blockade after myocardial infarction: systematic review and meta regression analysis, *Br Med J* 1999; **318**(7200): 1730–7.

28. Julian DG, Camm AJ, Frangin G et al, Randomised trial of effect of amiodarone on mortality in patients with left-ventricular dysfunction after recent myocardial infarction: EMIAT. European Myocardial Infarct Amiodarone Trial Investigators, *Lancet* 1997; **349**(9053): 667–74.

29. Cairns JA, Connolly SJ, Roberts R, Gent M, Randomised trial of outcome after myocardial infarction in patients with frequent or repetitive ventricular premature depolarisations: CAMIAT. Canadian Amiodarone Myocardial Infarction Arrhythmia Trial Investigators, *Lancet* 1997; **349**(9053): 675–82.

30. Amiodarone Trials Meta-Analysis Investigators, Effect of prophylactic amiodarone on mortality after acute myocardial infarction and in congestive heart failure: meta-analysis of individual data from 6500 patients in randomised trials, *Lancet* 1997; **350**(9089): 1417–24.

31. Waldo AL, Camm AJ, de Ruyter H et al, Effect of d-sotalol on mortality in patients with left ventricular dysfunction after recent and remote myocardial infarction. The SWORD Investigators. Survival With Oral d-Sotalol) *Lancet* 1996; **348**(9019): 7–12.

32. Danish Investigations of Arrhythmia and Mortality ON Dofetilide, Dofetilide in patients with left ventricular dysfunction and either heart failure or acute myocardial infarction: rationale, design, and patient characteristics of the DIAMOND studies, *Clin Cardiol* 1997; **20**(8): 704–10.

33. Camm AJ, Karam R, Pratt CM, The azimilide post-infarct survival evaluation (ALIVE) trial, *Am J Cardiol* 1998; **81**(6A): 35D–9D.

34. Moss AJ, Hall WJ, Cannom DS et al, Improved survival with an implanted defibrillator in patients with coronary disease at high risk for ventricular arrhythmia. Multicenter Automatic Defibrillator Implantation Trial Investigators, *N Engl J Med* 1996; **335**(26): 1933–40.

35. Nisam S, Mower M, ICD trials: an extraordinary means of determining patient risk? *Pacing Clin Electrophysiol* 1998; **21**(7): 1341–6.

Management of patients following discharge after myocardial infarction

Jason Pyatt and Paul Mullins

12

Introduction

Impressive improvements have occurred in both the diagnosis and management of acute myocardial infarction over recent years. Despite this, and the fall in the death rate from this disease, in the UK and elsewhere, it still remains one of the most important and feared of all illnesses.[1] Although the mortality has fallen, the prevalence of coronary artery disease and associated morbidity is increasing as populations are becoming more elderly. Those who survive to be discharged alive from hospital join the highest risk group for future cardiac events.

They have a 20-fold increase in the risk of coronary death over the next 10 years, and seven times the risk of reinfarction per year.[2] Over 70% of deaths from myocardial infarction occur outside hospital, and half of the patients include those who have had previous infarcts. Determining and modifying the risk of these preventable events in individual patients is crucial.

Fortunately, keeping patients in hospital for long periods is uncommon for uncomplicated patients, and they are often discharged at 5–10 days following admission. Patients are often aware of the worrying outlook and need to be motivated to modify things but maintain a decent quality of life.

There is a huge psychosocial and economic burden for society to bear, as myocardial infarction often strikes at the individual during their most productive time of life. In 1996, the estimated cost of coronary heart disease was approximately £5000 million in lost production.[3] Getting patients back to work if they are able is important for them as well as the Treasury. Another challenge is that the average age of the patients who have a myocardial infarction is increasing, and rehabilitation becomes more difficult, as many have other concurrent illnesses.

The main aim of the management of patients following discharge after myocardial infarction is to help alleviate patient symptoms, concerns and worries. Those at substantially increased risk of future ischaemic events need to be identified. Measures should be taken to slow the progression of underlying coronary heart disease through rehabilitation plus secondary prevention. The assessment of post-infarction prognosis and identifying those who may benefit from specific interventional therapies need to be identified. Translating the large amount of available research into patients

having an improved outcome and quality of life after surviving a heart attack is the main clinical challenge.

General advice

The psychological impact of having a myocardial infarction is huge. Anxiety is inevitably caused by the severe pain and then by the realization, usually for the first time, that they were facing death. Subsequently, they have to contend with the potential for prolonged disability or loss of employment. Not surprisingly, depression occurs in over 45% of patients following a myocardial infarction and is an independent risk factor for future increased mortality.[4] These concerns usually involve the patient's partner, family and friends. Early contact by the hospital with their general practitioner as well as a prompt discharge summary can do much to allay these worries. Uptake of lifestyle changes is poor and often ignored by those groups who are likely to benefit most. This can be addressed by several methods, including nurse-led prevention clinics and alternative information sources such as telephone 'hotlines'.

Patients are often told that it takes 4–6 weeks after their first myocardial infarction for the myocardium to 'heal'. Guidance should be started early, if appropriate, and booklets, videos, etc. can be useful. Patients should be

Table 12.1
Common patient anxieties after myocardial infarction.

> *What is going to happen to me in the future?*
> *What level of exercise should I do?*
> *What are the reasons for the heart attack?*
> *When can I resume having sexual intercourse?*
> *When can I start driving again?*
> *Should I stop smoking, and drinking alcohol?*
> *When can I start playing golf (etc.) again?*
> *What is going to happen at work if I go back?*

advised to expect some feelings of tiredness and general aches and pains in the immediate period after discharge. They should also be instructed on the use and side-effects of glyceryl trinitrate, and the other drugs they will take. They and their carers should be made aware of when and where to seek help if chest pains recur. In the era of thrombolytic and other acute treatments, they should be told to err on the side of caution. Specific guidance should be given and 'tailored' to each individual. Some relatives may want instruction on basic cardiopulmonary resuscitation. A team-based approach is usually necessary to meet these varying demands. The 'return to work' rate following a myocardial infarction is up to 90%.[5]

However, these relatively high rates are to some extent offset by many patients who retire or are made redundant in the medium term. Some are disbarred from work, such as airline pilots, lorry drivers, and bus and coach drivers. Others, whose occupations involve heavy manual work, simply cannot perform their job.

Unfortunately, guidelines on returning to employment do not exist for the majority of occupations. Confusion can arise between patient and medical advisor as to what constitutes a safe level of physical activity and the timing of any subsequent return. Exercise ECG testing is useful and this is discussed later in this chapter. The average time taken to return to work is 60–70 days but patients often subsequently report reduced earnings and increased work-related stress.

Table 12.2
Factors involved in returning to work after myocardial infarction.

> *Age*
> *Occupation*
> *Number of previous myocardial infarctions*
> *Other chronic illnesses*
> *Patient's, relatives' and employers' attitudes to myocardial infarction*
> *Proximity to retirement age*
> *Driving status*
> *Medication*

Sexual activity

Common sexual problems after myocardial infarction include reduced libido, impotence, chest pains, premature or delayed ejaculation in men and the fear of provoking a cardiac event. Some of these are caused by pre-existing sexual dysfunction, depression and the result of drug therapy—especially beta-blockers and diuretics. Patients and partners can be reassured that the haemodynamic response to sexual intercourse in those recovering from myocardial infarction is normally less than that attained during an exercise test. However, this response is far greater in unusual surroundings, after heavy meals, with the consumption of alcohol, and with unfamiliar partners.[6] It will be interesting to see the impact of the new agents aimed as a treatment for male impotence, such as Viagra, if their use becomes widespread. Viagra's use within 6 months of a heart attack is not recommended at the moment, and it can potentiate the hypotensive effect of nitrates.

Exercise testing can be used to predict the likelihood of developing cardiac stress as a result of sexual activity, and those with significant abnormalities on treadmill testing can be advised to resume their sexual activity gradually. In general, most patients are advised that it is safe to resume love-making at about 4 weeks after a heart attack, if their partner will let them! Many patients and their loved one find it difficult to volunteer information about sexual problems. Medical staff can do much to allay these fears. This includes inviting open discussion and providing information to patients and their partners, using booklets and other methods. They should be told to report symptoms such as angina, excessive breathlessness or palpitations (tachycardia) lasting 10 min after intercourse. These may be the only manifestations of residual ischaemia or left ventricular dysfunction.

Driving and travel

The ordinary car driver is usually advised not to drive for 4 weeks after an uncomplicated myocardial infarction. Patients with certain arrhythmias, and employees who drive a vehicle for a living, such as lorry drivers and bus drivers, require special assessment before being allowed to return to work. This is mainly guided by the Driving Vehicle Licensing Authority (DVLA) regulations. Taxi drivers usually have to comply with local guidance by their licensing authority. The contact address to obtain the up-to-date regulations is The Medical Officer, DVLA, Swansea, SA99 1BN.

It seems sensible to advise against travel abroad until after patients have been reviewed as outpatients at approximately 6 weeks post-infarction. Even then, travel may have to be further delayed if they are still symptomatic or awaiting investigations. Common sense is usually the best guide.

Cardiac rehabilitation

The role of cardiac rehabilitation is to help patients get back to a normal or as near normal a life as possible following a myocardial infarction.[7] The process begins early after the onset of the heart attack and involves an integrated approach combining education, counselling, lifestyle modification and exercise training.[8] Rehabilitation efforts used to be mainly directed at those who had made a good physical recovery from their infarction. However, such patients are at relatively low risk and suffer more from anxiety and depression than from physical disability. It is accepted now that patients with heart failure and angina can also benefit from rehabilitation, especially if it is centred on physical training.

The evaluation of the efficacy of cardiac rehabilitation has concentrated on overviews of exercise-based rehabilitation, purely psychological rehabilitation, and comprehensive programmes amalgamating all aspects of rehabilitation. These trials are strongly influenced by patient selection, the end-points used, and the difficulties of combining multiple small trials of low statistical power and markedly variable results.

Even so, these statistical overviews suggest a mortality benefit from all types of rehabilitation at least comparable to those gained by pharmacological secondary prevention methods. For example, the pooling of 10 trials using exercise training showed a significant (22%) reduction in mortality.[9] Despite these undoubted benefits, the provision and uptake rates following invitation to rehabilitation are poor. Regular assessment of the use of these services should be undertaken.[10]

In another example of the 'inverse care law', patients from low socio-economic groups have the highest risk of developing further coronary artery disease events but the lowest attendance rates. Women are also poor attenders, possibly because they have to do more things at home than men! Community-based cardiac rehabilitation programmes may help in achieving greater compliance and are associated with success and complication rates comparable to those of hospital-based ones. Proposed changes in government funding may support effective development in rehabilitation services.[11]

Risk assessment

It is important to identify at an early stage those patients who are at high risk for future cardiac events.[12] Many of these risks can be modified. Some may be candidates for interventional therapies such as coronary artery bypass grafting, or percutaneous coronary angioplasty, to reduce that risk further. The previous emphasis on only performing these invasive investigations and treatments on young, symptomatic or very symptomatic elderly patients has fortunately changed. The basis of this risk stratification is to identify the 'high-risk' patients who are suitable whatever their age. It should commence during their hospital stay and continue beyond the time of hospital discharge. The influences on choosing who gets the 'invasive' approach are not always straightforward. The amount of service provision versus demand is often a critical factor. These various investigations may provide a guide on the degree of ventricular impairment, the presence of residual

ischaemia and the tendency to develop complex ventricular arrhythmia. Some factors can influence patient outcome.

The treadmill exercise ECG test is the most widely used and probably the most validated way to predict risk on recovery after myocardial infarction.[13] This is despite the relatively recent introduction of thrombolytic treatment, and suggestions that it is now less helpful. It can provide information on the presence and extent of any underlying residual ischaemia, ventricular function and arrhythmias as well. It is also an independent risk predictor if other variables are taken into account. About a third of patients cannot perform an exercise test and have the worst prognosis of all.

There is no need to discontinue beta-blockers prior to exercise testing, as most of the original data concerning the test and prognosis after myocardial infarction were obtained in patients already receiving them. There is also a clinical risk in stopping these drugs quickly.

The risk of complications arising when performing submaximal exercise ECG testing before hospital discharge is higher, but picks out those with the worse prognosis early. Alternatively, a maximal exercise test may be performed 6 weeks after discharge, with less complications, but misses some of the sickest

Table 12.3
Variables predicting poorer prognosis after myocardial infarction.

Increasing age
Female gender
Poor residual left ventricular function
Previous myocardial infarction
Patency of the infarct-related artery
Multiple coronary risk factors
Extent of the underlying coronary
    disease
Significant arrhythmias
Hypertension
Diabetes mellitus
Poorer socio-economic class

patients. The resources available often determine what happens in each hospital.

Some features indicate a poorer prognosis and suggest the need for invasive investigations and treatment.

ST segment depression may not always be present as a predictor of prognosis in those who have exercise capacity impaired by poor left ventricular function. Angina and ST segment depression during a post-discharge test increase the likelihood of chronic angina. Asymptomatic ST depression is associated with a 12-fold increase in mortality compared with a negative test.[14] ST segment elevation seen in leads where Q-waves are present probably indicates an underlying dyskinetic segment of myocardium, whereas in a non-Q-wave lead, it implies a high probability of critical residual ischaemia. Unfortunately, treating the latter group invasively is still not of clear benefit prognostically.

In those patients unable to exercise, or with

baseline electrocardiographic abnormalities which make accurate interpretation during exercise difficult (e.g. left bundle branch block), radioisotope myocardial perfusion scanning,[15] or possibly stress echocardiography, are the main alternative means of assessing risk. Although more technically demanding, and expensive, both are more sensitive and specific than exercise electrocardiography.

Residual left ventricular function is the main determinant of outcome in myocardial infarction patients. The role of routine echocardiography in these patients is expanding, particularly as many asymptomatic patients have poor left ventricles. Either this or the use of radioisotopic MUGA (multi-gated acquisition) scanning to assess left ventricular function should become more widespread to detect and monitor this, often asymptomatic, situation.

There is some debate about using coronary angiography in every patient post-myocardial

Table 12.4
Predictors of poor outcome on exercise ECG testing after myocardial infarction.

> *Onset of angina*
> *Electrocardiographic evidence of ischaemia (> 1 mm ST segment depression)*
> *Drop in systolic blood pressure (> 10 mmHg) compared to rest*
> *Failure to reach target heart rate*
> *Significant arrhythmias (e.g. ventricular tachycardia, ventricular fibrillation)*

infarction. This would have the advantage of providing an instantaneous anatomical picture of the coronary arterial lumen, and the number and severity of large stenoses, if present. However, the functional significance of the lesions would be missing, and the majority of infarcts occur from ruptured coronary arterial plaques with associated thrombus. The majority of these are less than 50% of adjacent arterial diameter prior to rupture, and are hard to detect.[16] They may not cause much in the way of preceding angina symptoms. The proportion of patients with significant coronary artery disease who may be suitable from a prognostic perspective post-myocardial infarction, is dependent on the group of patients studied. However, roughly, 25–30% of patients have three-vessel coronary artery disease, or proximal left anterior lesions and another vessel, while only 1–2% have 'left main' coronary disease. The rest have one- and two-vessel disease, which do not improve in prognosis with intervention and are treated only if symptomatic. Results from recent studies of aggressive percutaneous intervention in all patients early after infarction have not shown a survival advantage over those treated conservatively.[17] Most centres in the UK use cardiac catheterization only in selected patients post-myocardial infarction.

To conclude, the role of investigations is to treat symptomatic patients, detect those with a poor prognosis and intervene where appropriate. Patients need to be made aware of the risks versus benefits: high-technology treatments are not always the best thing for many patients.

Secondary prevention

Secondary prevention is defined as the prevention of the progression of symptomatic coronary heart disease. In those patients discharged following a myocardial infarction, this translates into a reduction in the rate of reinfarction, angina, heart failure and death. The same risk factors that contribute to the initial development of coronary heart disease events also predict their recurrence. It is of vital importance to try and get things right— approximately half the patients who die are already known to have coronary heart disease. As the absolute risk of further events is so much higher compared with the general population, far fewer patients need to be treated to save one life or prevent one clinical event, making it a much more cost-effective strategy than primary prevention. In addition, the various risk factors interact in a multiplicative rather than an additive way to predict poor outcome.

There is now good evidence from randomized prospective trials that some forms of lifestyle modification and many adjunctive drug treatments can have a significant impact in

Table 12.5
Risk factors and risk of subsequent coronary event.

40-year-old male with no other risks	
40-year-old male hypertensive	••
40-year-old male smoker	••
40-year-old male with hypercholesterolaemia	•••
40-year-old male smoker with hypertension and hypercholesterolaemia	••••••

•, Risk of coronary heart disease events compared to baseline patient.

improving prognosis post-myocardial infarction. Despite these benefits, the use of these preventative measures has been variable for both doctors and patients. Of even more concern is the extensive usage of agents that do not improve prognosis or even may actually do harm, such as some calcium-channel blockers or anti-arrhythmic drugs (see below). To assess how risk factors are recorded in clinical practice and the implementation of secondary prevention, a survey termed ASPIRE (Action on Secondary Prevention through Intervention to Reduce Events) was undertaken by the British Cardiac Society at numerous hospitals throughout the UK during 1994 and 1995.[18] This showed that the documentation, the treatment of certain conditions and the use of prophylactic drug therapy was poor. For example, 25% of patients had untreated diastolic hypertension, 40% had no record of their total cholesterol, and beta-blocker prescription was present in only 38%.

Hospitals need to perform regular 'in-house' audits, create standardized admission plus treatment protocols, and adopt other measures to address these issues. Support for a strong community-based programme could make an important difference.[19]

Non-pharmacological

Smoking
Smoking is a strong risk factor for a first myocardial infarction and for fatal and non-fatal recurrences. Observational trials have shown that smoking cessation is associated with a 50% reduction in mortality rate over 2 years of follow-up.[20] Stopping smoking delays the onset of angina after myocardial infarction, making it one of the most effective forms of secondary prevention. Most patients stop smoking immediately after a heart attack and appear receptive to advice about lifestyle measures. Unfortunately, a return to old habits is common and continued support is

vital. Nicotine replacement therapy doubles the number of those who stop smoking for 6–12 months. Those who stop smoking after a week's treatment do best overall, and this may be a guide as to how long to try this therapy.[21] Caution is necessary in using it soon after discharge from hospital.

Diet and obesity

Although there is no trial evidence showing a change in prognosis, obesity is often related to a poor diet, and is associated with hypertension and other problems. A weight-reducing diet is appropriate, particularly for those who are overweight (body mass index, BMI >25) or obese (BMI >30). To calculate BMI, divide the weight in kilograms by the height in metres squared. The former group have double the risk of heart disease, while the latter face a quadrupled risk, and some diets may reduce this.[22] All post-infarction patients should adopt a diet rich in fruit and vegetables and low in saturated fat. Combining diet with exercise is still the main way of losing weight. Weight-reducing drugs should be avoided at present.

Exercise

All post-myocardial infarction patients should be given specific advice concerning physical activity. This needs to be tailored to the needs of each patient, taking into account age, pre-existing fitness and coincident disabilities. This is aided by supervised increasing walking and other activities on the wards. An exercise ECG test helps and often forms part of a formal cardiac rehabilitation programme. An overview of 22 randomized trials of exercise rehabilitation following infarction showed that cardiovascular mortality was reduced by 20% and fatal reinfarction by 25% over 3 years of follow-up.[23] On average, patients with coronary heart disease and no contraindications should be encouraged to undertake regular aerobic exercise for 20–30 min at a time at least three times a week.

Unfortunately, there are large areas of the country that do not have any formal rehabilitation schemes, and many patients do not attend if there is one. Coordination needs to be improved between patients, general practitioners, hospitals and possibly national rehabilitation networks. The British Heart Foundation is developing a nurse-based scheme and there are similar schemes with charity or other funding throughout the country.

Alcohol

Moderate levels of alcohol consumption appear to exert a cardioprotective effect.[24] This is probably mediated directly, through a reduction in plasma fibrinogen levels and through increased high-density lipoprotein (HDL) subfractions of lipoproteins creating a decreased risk of myocardial infarction.

Against this, increasing intake can negate this benefit by increasing systolic blood pressure,[25] obesity, and the risk of sudden death. As a personal observation, confirmed by others, it is more likely that people will resume smoking if they are in the pub. They should be encouraged to go into a 'no smoking section' if there is one. There are varying guidelines about what constitute modest quantities of alcohol. Let us hope that the old 'definition' of an alcoholic as someone who drinks more than his doctor is still untrue!

Hypertension
There is evidence that hypertensive patients do worse than normotensive patients after myocardial infarction.[26] There are no trials, as placing a control group on placebo would be unethical. Both beta-blockers and ACE inhibitors are given to most patients, and fortunately lower the blood pressure.

Diabetes mellitus
Coronary heart disease is a major complication for both type 1 and type 2 diabetes, and risk is increased post-myocardial infarction. In the Framingham study, the risk of reinfarction was increased by 50% and the long-term mortality was doubled in post-myocardial infarction diabetic patients compared with non-diabetics.[26] Diabetic patients are also more likely to have hypertension, obesity and abnormal lipid profiles. All patients, following a heart attack,

should be screened for diabetes. Although no studies have shown tight glycaemic control to reduce macrovascular complications, studies have shown combined strict blood pressure control and good glycaemic control to be beneficial.

Pharmacological

Antiplatelet and anticoagulant agents
Aspirin is established as a proven, effective and relatively safe therapy for both the treatment of myocardial infarction and its secondary prevention. The Antiplatelet Trialists' Collaboration meta-analysis showed a 25% reduction in the risk of recurrent infarction and death in post-infarct patients given daily doses of aspirin between 80 and 325 mg.[27] When a myocardial infarction occurs in those already taking aspirin, it appears to be smaller in size and often non-Q-wave in nature. Aspirin should be prescribed to those who can tolerate it immediately after the onset of symptoms and carried on indefinitely. Ensuring that patients are prescribed and continue to take aspirin is important. In a community-based study, a multidisciplinary scheme increased aspirin prescription from under 50% to nearly 90% of appropriate patients.[28] Alternative antiplatelet agents such as dipyridamole and clopidigrel should be considered for those who cannot tolerate aspirin, although the evidence is much less clear.

Oral anticoagulants are also effective in reducing reinfarction and death in survivors of myocardial infarction, but the data are from patients in trials conducted prior to the introduction of thrombolytic therapy and the anticoagulation was commenced at least 2 weeks after the index event. In later trials, the evidence was less conclusive and direct comparisons with antiplatelet agents showed neither clear-cut cost-effective benefit nor superior clinical efficacy. Patients with specific clinical abnormalities such as left ventricular aneurysm, atrial fibrillation or mural thrombus seen on echocardiography do appear to benefit from early oral anticoagulants, but, again, evidence from large, randomized studies is lacking.

The use of low-dose anticoagulation with aspirin after thrombolysis showed no benefit.[29] The results of other trials addressing the use of anticoagulant versus aspirin, outpatient early use of subcutaneous heparins, and oral glycoprotein IIb/IIa receptor antagonists plus others, are eagerly awaited.

Beta-adrenergic antagonist drugs

Drugs with beta-adrenergic receptor antagonist properties (beta-blockers) have anti-arrhythmic, anti-ischaemic and antihypertensive effects. Given to patients with myocardial infarction, they can reduce chest pain, myocardial wall stress and infarct size. They can reduce mortality by 13% when administered during the first few hours after infarction. Oral beta-blockers started 5–28 days post-myocardial infarction can significantly reduce mortality for at least 2–3 years. In the Norwegian Multicentre Study, timolol, at a dose of 5 or 10 mg twice daily, 7–28 days after infarction, reduced the risk of reinfarction by 28% and overall mortality by 39% at 33 months.[30] These benefits persisted for up to 6 years. Similar results have been seen in other studies.[31] These positive findings are apparent among all subgroups analysed, and serious side-effects are few. Unfortunately, as noted above in the ASPIRE study and others, these agents are underused in the UK. Another aspect is that since intravenous beta-blockers post-myocardial infarction reduce the amount of myocardial damage, those already on these agents, with satisfactory serum levels, may benefit if they have a further infarct. Therefore, beta-blockers should be prescribed to all relevant patients after myocardial infarction who do not have definite contraindications and, if tolerated, continued indefinitely.

Angiotensin-converting enzyme inhibitors

As noted previously, impaired left ventricular function is the main determinant of outcome for post-myocardial infarction patients. The angiotensin-converting enzyme (ACE) inhibitors have a favourable impact on adverse left ventricular remodelling after myocardial infarction and slow progression to subsequent congestive heart failure. Evidence for decreased mortality in post-myocardial infarction patients, particularly those with left ventricular dysfunction, comes from several studies.[32] Randomized trial evidence has shown the largest mortality benefit in those patients started on early treatment after the patient is stable, and most of all in those with large infarcts and left ventricular impairment.

Some of those trials, representative of what is seen in clinical practice, are shown in Table 12.6.

Recent further analysis of patients included in the original AIRE study (AIREX) and other evidence supports the continued use of ACE inhibitors in the long term.[39] Patients with

Table 12.6
Trials of ACE inhibitors given to patients post-myocardial infarction.

Title	Patients	Drugs	Time started post-myocardial infarction	Follow-up	One-year mortality in treated group (%)	Mortality RR (%)
SAVE[33]	Asymptomatic EF<40%	High-dose captopril up to 50 mg tds	3–16 days 3–11 days	2–5 years	10	19
AIRE[34]	Clinical heart failure	Moderate-dose myocardial infarction up to 5 mg bd		6–30 months	16	27
TRACE[35]	EF<35%	Trandolapril up to 4 mg od	3–7 days	2–4 years	24	22
SMILE[36]	Anterior myocardial infarction without thrombolysis	Zofenopril up to 30 mg od for 4 weeks	<24 h	Up to 1 year	14	29
GISSI-3[37]	All patients without contraindication	Lisinopril up to 10 mg od for 6 weeks	<24 h	Up to 6 months	N/A	11
ISIS 4[38]	All patients without contraindication	Captopril up to 50 mg bd for 6 weeks	<24 h	Up to 6 months	N/A	7
CONSENSUS II[39]	All patients without contraindication	Intravenous enalaprilat over 2 h and oral enalapril up to 20 mg bd	<24 h	Up to 6 months	N/A	None seen

EF, ejection fraction; relative risk.

signs of left ventricular dysfunction post-myocardial infarction, whether symptomatic or not, should be prescribed ACE inhibitors for at least 3 years.

Another contentious issue is whether the lower doses of these agents which are commonly used in clinical practice are as effective as the higher ones used in clinical trials. A recent, as yet unpublished, study, the ATLAS trial, was presented at the 47th Annual American College of Cardiology Scientific Meeting in May 1998. An investigation of the use of lisinopril at 2.5–5 mg od (low dose) or 32.5–35 mg od (high dose) in heart failure showed that higher doses in patients who can tolerate them produced a significant reduction in combined all-cause mortality and hospitalization (12%). This approach is probably the best one to use for all agents.

The best clinical approach is to treat patients as soon as they are stable. Treatment should definitely be given to those with evidence of heart failure, large infarcts, anterior infarcts, and previous infarcts. Drug dose should be increased to the maximum tolerated clinically, and prescribed indefinitely. Those with any suspicion of 'occult' left ventricular dysfunction at any stage, particularly patients with inferior myocardial infarcts who are not doing as well as they should, should be investigated The routine use of

echocardiography or radioisotope multi-gated acquisition scan (MUGA) to assess and monitor all post-myocardial infarction patients would be ideal, but resources are often limited.

Preliminary studies of the newer angiotensin II receptor antagonists (e.g. losartan, valsartan) in patients with heart failure have been encouraging, but their role in post-myocardial infarction patients is not clear.

HMG-CoA reductase inhibitors
Hyperlidaemia is strongly linked to coronary artery disease both as an initiating factor and in its subsequent progression. Atherosclerotic plaques mainly consist of arterial wall tissue, inflammatory cells, and varying amounts of connective tissue and lipids. The softer the plaque, mainly if it contains a lot of lipid, the more likely it is to rupture. Low-density lipoprotein (LDL) cholesterol, a subfraction of total cholesterol, has the strongest association with coronary disease.

The use of lipid-lowering agents was problematic until the development of newer agents. The role of the powerful cholesterol-lowering drugs (the 'statins') in secondary prevention has become much clearer with the publication of several major randomized, controlled, clinical trials. The main studies in post-myocardial infarction patients are shown in Table 12.7.

Table 12.7
Trials of 'statins' used after myocardial infarction.

Title	Patients	Drugs	Cholesterol	Mortality RR (%)
4S[40]	Post-myocardial infarction or angina for median of 5.4 years	20–40 mg od simvastatin	'High' total cholesterol, 5.5–8.0 mmol/l	30
CARE[41]	Post-myocardial infarction for 5 years	Pravastatin 40 mg daily	'Normal' total cholesterol–mean total cholesterol 5.4 mmol/L	24
LIPID[42]	Post-myocardial infarction for 6 years	Pravastatin 40 mg daily	'Usual' range of total cholesterol 4–7 mmol/l	22

A consistent reduction of about a third in the risk of stroke was also seen in these studies. The main message is that post-myocardial infarction patients are more likely to benefit from these agents than many others, as their risk of future cardiac events is so high. The latest European guidelines suggest treatment for total cholesterol of 5.0 mmol/l, and LDL cholesterol <3.0 mmol/l.[43] There is a case for starting all post-myocardial infarction patients on statins, but the evidence for this is controversial. Assessment of baseline risk for patients in primary prevention to determine whether drugs should be given may be helpful. Various guidelines have suggested that these patients should have an annual risk of cardiac events of 2–3% before treatment is started.[44] These issues have not been settled in primary prevention, but the prescribing threshold in post-infarction patients should be low. One aspect of this is cost. However, treating those patients was very cost-effective, at £5000 per life year saved. The drug dosage should probably be adjusted to produce at least a 30% reduction in the baseline LDL cholesterol level.

The treatment of other lipid subfraction abnormalities such as hypertriglyceridaemia are less well established. The use of other drugs such as resin binding agents (cholestyramine, etc.), nicotinic acid and fibrates is not as well supported by trials, but may be necessary in the rare patients who cannot tolerate statins.

Calcium-channel blocking drugs, nitrates and magnesium

Despite their anti-anginal, vasodilatory and antihypertensive properties, calcium-channel antagonists have not yet been clearly shown to reduce mortality when administered during or after myocardial infarction in either individual trials or meta-analyses.[45] The older, short-acting dihydropyridines at high dosages appear to be potentially hazardous, and all agents should be used cautiously in patients with poor left ventricular function. Some of the newer, longer-acting dihydropyridines, which are less negatively inotropic (e.g. amlodipine), appear to have a neutral effect when used in heart failure patients.

Verapamil, given post-myocardial infarction, produced a 20% reduction in death and reinfarction but only if left ventricular function was good.[46] A subgroup analysis of diltiazem used after infarction in patients without pulmonary congestion showed that it reduced cardiac events by 23%. Those with pulmonary congestion had an increased event rate.[47]

One of the latest of a new class of these agents, mibefradil, was withdrawn after its introduction, as it interacted with drugs that cardiac patients were also likely to take. Current evidence is against a role for calcium antagonists in post-infarction secondary prevention, and their usage should be restricted to symptom relief and to improve exercise tolerance.

The use of nitrates and intravenous magnesium sulphate did not make a significant impact in the large ISIS-4 study which included them in its design.[38]

Anti-arrhythmic agents

Up to 52% of sudden cardiac death victims are found to have evidence of prior infarction at autopsy. Patients with frequent ventricular premature beats after infarction have a fourfold increase in mortality rate. Attempts to suppress these prophylactically with class 1 agents increase mortality (Cardiac Arrhythmia Suppression Trial—CAST).[48] This and other studies showed a significant (21%) increase in death rate.[49]

Both sotalol and amiodarone have class 3 properties and are theoretically attractive for reducing arrhythmias and sudden death post-myocardial infarction. I-Sotalol had a neutral effect on sudden death in post-infarct patients. A large trial using the 'pure' class 3 agent, *d*-sotalol, was terminated prematurely due to excess mortality in those on active treatment.[50]

Two of the latest large trials involving amiodarone routinely after myocardial infarction have produced less than encouraging results. The Canadian Amiodarone Myocardial Infarction Trial

(CAMIAT) showed reduced arrhythmic death and resuscitation from ventricular fibrillation, but 42% stopped the drug due to intolerable side-effects.[51] The European Myocardial Infarction Trial (EMIAT) showed only a reduction in arrhythmic death in patients with depressed left ventricular function, but overall mortality remained unchanged.[52]

At the present time, the routine use of anti-arrhythmic agents post myocardial infarction cannot be recommended.

'Rough guide' to benefits of post-myocardial infarction treatment

The relative risk reductions comparing the risk of treated groups versus the control group have been used throughout the chapter so far.

Absolute risk reductions are a valid attempt to compare the risk of an event in groups in a way that is clear. Obviously, there are limitations, as the studies have all been in groups with different baseline risk and therefore should be interpreted with caution.

However, absolute risk is often easier for patients (and others!) to understand, using concepts such as the effect of treatment per 1000 patient years. For example, suggesting that a room is full of 200 patients after a myocardial infarction, and at the end of 5 years the lucky ones meet again to find out what has happened that could have been avoided, can be useful. It is best to avoid the question about how to be one of those patients who do not do anything and still get away with it! A few examples of effect on mortality taken from several studies are shown in Table 12.8.

Table 12.8
Effect of intervention as deaths prevented per 1000 patient years.

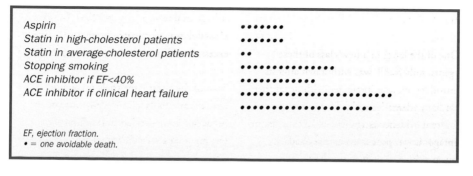

Aspirin	•••••••
Statin in high-cholesterol patients	•••••••
Statin in average-cholesterol patients	••
Stopping smoking	••••••••••••••
ACE inhibitor if EF<40%	••••••••••••
ACE inhibitor if clinical heart failure	•••

EF, ejection fraction.
• = one avoidable death.

Possible future treatments

The benefits of the use of hormone replacement treatment in postmenopausal women to prevent coronary disease are not clear. Most of the encouraging studies have been observational studies, and biased towards healthier women taking this treatment and consequently having less cardiac disease. Prospective controlled studies are being performed. It is important to note that the use of these agents is not contraindicated in women after acute myocardial infarction.[53]

As mentioned previously, the use of subcutaneous low molecular weight heparins given for an extensive period after discharge is being evaluated. Drugs which act on other parts of the thrombosis pathway are undergoing trial.

The role of diet in reducing cardiac events is unclear. There are suggestions that the use of dietary and pharmacological antioxidants,[54] such as oral, high-dose, vitamin E, may be useful. Newer anti-anginal agents which are becoming available, such as nicorandil,[55] may also offer new pharmacological benefits to post-myocardial infarction patients.

The intriguing suggestion that coronary artery disease might be due to microbial infection has been extensively reinvestigated, partly stimulated by the revelation that most duodenal ulcers are associated with *Helicobacter pylori* infection. This particular organism is unlikely to cause arterial disease, but treatment of *Chlamydia pneumoniae* in acute unstable coronary syndromes is being thoroughly investigated.[56] Could antibiotics put coronary care units out of business?

Conclusion

Much can be done to improve the outcome and wellbeing of the fortunate patients following their discharge from hospital after a myocardial infarction. Practical advice on such issues as returning to work or driving is often overlooked but is immensely important to the patient. Enrollment in a formal cardiac rehabilitation programme aids recovery, and exercise training in particular is beneficial.

Risk stratification should be performed by close clinical evaluation coupled with the careful use of further investigations. Identifying those who may benefit from selective treatment and reassuring those at low risk is important, and needs to be improved. Secondary preventative measures involving either lifestyle changes or prophylactic drug therapies are effective in reducing the heavy toll of future coronary events. We need to let patients be involved in the many decisions necessary in recovering from a heart attack, but also make sure they have the best quality of life possible.

These patients now act as a risk factor for developing coronary disease for their families. It is important to make sure they pass on what they have learned from their myocardial infarction, and to get them to set a good example.

References

1. San S, Kestelloo, Kromhout D, on behalf of the Task Force of the European Society of Cardiology in Cardiovascular Mortality and Morbidity Statistics in Europe, The burden of cardiovascular diseases mortality in Europe, *Eur Heart J* 1997; **18:** 1231–48.

2. Shaper AG, Pocock SJ, Walker M et al, Risk factors for ischaemic heart disease: the prospective phase of the British Regional Heart Study, *J Epidemiol Community Health* 1985; **39:** 197–209.

3. Coronary heart disease statistics book 1997, British Heart Foundation, 14 Fitzhardinge Street, London W1H 4DH.

4. Schleifer SJ, Macari-Hinson MM, Coyle DA et al, The nature and course of depression following myocardial infarction, *Arch Intern Med* 1989; **149:** 1785–9.

5. Smith GR, O'Rourke DF, Return to work after myocardial infarction: a test of multiple hypotheses, *JAMA* 1988; **259:** 1673–7.

6. Goodman R, Sex counselling for the post-coronary patient, *Cardiol Practice* 1990; **8:** 14–16.

7. Norris RM, Barnaby PF, Brandt PWT et al, Prognosis after recovery from first myocardial infarction: determinants of reinfarction and sudden death, *Am J Cardiol* 1984; **53:** 408–11.

8. Horgan J, Bethell H, Carson P et al, Working party report on cardiac rehabilitation, *Br Heart J* 1992; **67:** 412–18.

9. Oldbridge NB, Guyatt GH, Fischer MD, Rimm AA, Cardiac rehabilitation after myocardial infarction: combined experience of randomised clinical trials, *JAMA* 1988; **260:** 945–50.

10. Thompson DR, Bowman GS, Kitson AL, De Bono DP, Cardiac rehabilitation: guidelines and audit standards, *Heart* 1996; **75:** 89–93.

11. De Bono DP, Models of cardiac rehabilitation, *Br Med J* 1998; **316:** 1329–30.

12. ACC\AHA Task Force on Early Management of Acute Myocardial Infarction: Guidelines for the early management of patients with acute myocardial infarction, *J Am Coll Cardiol* 1990; **16:** 249–61.

13. Jennings K, Reid DS, Hawkins T, Julian DJ, Role of exercise testing early after myocardial infarction in identifying candidates for surgery, *Br Med J Clin Res* 1984; **288:** 185–7.

14. De Belder M, Skehan D, Pumphrey C et al, Identification of a high risk subgroup of patients with silent ischaemia after myocardial infarction: a group for early therapeutic revascularisation? *Br Heart J* 1990; **63:** 145–50.

15. Gibson RS, Beller GA, Value of predischarge myocardial perfusion scintigraphy. In: Foster V, Ross R, Topol EJ, eds, *Atherosclerosis and Coronary Artery Disease* (Lippincott-Raven: Philadelphia, 1996) 1167–92.

16. Little WC, Constantinescu MS, Applegate RJ et al, Can coronary angiography predict site of subsequent myocardial infarction in patients with mild to moderate coronary artery disease? *Circulation* 1988; **78:** 1157–66.

17. Williams DO, Braunwald E, Knatterud G

et al, One year results of the thrombolysis in myocardial infarction investigation (TIMI) phase 11 trial, *Circulation* 1992; **85:** 533–42.

18. Bowker TJ, Clayton TC, Ingham J et al, A British Cardiac Society survey of the potential for the secondary prevention of coronary disease—ASPIRE, *Heart* 1996; **75:** 334–42.

19. Campbell NC, Thain J, Deans G et al, Secondary prevention clinics for coronary heart disease: randomised trial of effect on health, *Br Med J* 1998; **316:** 1434–7.

20. Wilhelmsson C, Vedin A, Elmfeldt D et al, Smoking and myocardial infarction, *Lancet* 1975; **i:** 415–20.

21. Yudkin PL, Jones L, Lancaster T, Fowler GH, Which smokers are helped to give up smoking using transdermal nicotine patches? Results from a randomized, double blind, placebo controlled trial, *Br J Gen Pract* 1996; **46:** 145–8.

22. Burr ML, Fehily AM, Gilbert JF et al, Effects of changes in fat, fish, and fibre intakes on death and reinfarction. Diet and reinfarction trial, *Lancet* 1989; **ii:** 757–61.

23. O'Connor GT, Buring JE, Yusef S et al, An overview of randomised trials of rehabilitation with exercise after myocardial infarction, *Circulation* 1989; **80:** 234–44.

24. Rimm EB, Klatsky A, Grobbee D, Stampfer MJ, Review of moderate alcohol consumption and reduced risk of coronary heart disease: is the effect due to beer, wine or spirits? *Br Med J* 1996; **312:** 731–6.

25. Kannel WB, Sorlie P, Hypertension in Framingham. In: Paul O, ed., *Epidemiology and Control of Hypertension* (Stratton: New York, 1975) 553–92.

26. Wong ND, Cupples LA, Ostfeld AM et al, Risk factors for long-term coronary prognosis after initial myocardial infarction: The Framingham Study, *Am J Epidemiol* 1989; **138:** 469–80.

27. Antiplatelet Trialists' Collaboration, Collaborative overview of randomised trials of antiplatelet therapy—I: prevention of death, myocardial infarction, and stroke by prolonged antiplatelet therapy in various categories of patients, *Br Med J* 1994; **308:** 81–106.

28. The Liverpool Aspirin Project, *Putting Evidence in to Practice* (Liverpool Primary Care Audit Group: Liverpool, 1997).

29. Julian DG, Chamberlain DA, Pocock SJ for the AFTER Study Group, A comparison of aspirin and anticoagulation following thrombolysis for myocardial infarction (the AFTER study): a multicentre unblinded randomised clinical trial, *Br Med J* 1996; **313:** 1429–31.

30. The Norwegian Multicenter Study Group, Timolol-induced reduction in mortality and reinfarction in patients surviving acute myocardial infarction, *N Engl J Med* 1981; **304:** 801–7.

31. Teo KK, Yusuf S, Furberg CD, Effects of prophylactic antiarrhythmic drug therapy in acute myocardial infarction: an overview of results from randomised controlled trials, *JAMA* 1993; **270:** 1589–95.

32. Latini R, Maggioni A, Flather M et al, For the meeting participants. ACE inhibitor use in patients with myocardial infarction: summary of evidence from clinical trials, *Circulation* 1995; **92:** 3132–7.

33. Pfeffer MA, Braunwald E, Moye LA et al, Effect of captopril on mortality and morbidity in patients with left ventricular dysfunction after myocardial infarction, *N Engl J Med* 1992; **327:** 669–77.

34. The Acute Infarction Ramipril Efficacy (AIRE) Study Investigators, Effect of ramipril on mortality and morbidity of survivors of acute myocardial infarction with clinical evidence of heart failure, *Lancet* 1993; **342:** 821–8.

35. Kober L, Torp-Pederson C, Carlsen JE et al, A clinical trial of the angiotensin-converting-enzyme inhibitor trandolapril in patients with left ventricular dysfunction after myocardial infarction, *N Engl J Med* 1995; **333:** 1670–6.

36. Ambrosioni E, Borghi C, Magani B, Survival of Myocardial Infarction Long term Evaluation (SMILE) study, *Controlled Clin Trials* 1994; **15:** 201–19.

37. Third Gruppo Italiano per lo Studio della Sopravivenza nell' Infarcto miocardio (GISSI 3), Effects of lisinopril and transdermal glyceryl trinitrate singularly and together on six week mortality and ventricular function after myocardial infarction, *Lancet* 1994; **343:** 1115–22.

38. ISIS-4 (Fourth International Study on Infarct Survival) Collaborative Group, A randomised factorial trial assessing early oral captopril, oral mononitrate, and intravenous magnesium sulphate in 58,050 patients with suspected acute myocardial infarction, *Lancet* 1995; **345:** 990–5.

39. Hall AS, Murray GD, Ball SG et al, Follow up study of patients randomly allocated ramipril or placebo for heart failure after acute myocardial infarction: AIRE Extension (AIREX) Study, *Lancet* 1997; **349:** 1493–7.

40. Scandinavian Simvastatin Survival Study Group, Randomised trial of cholesterol lowering in 4444 patients with coronary heart disease: the Scandinavian Simvastatin Survival Study (4S), *Lancet* 1994; **344:** 1383–9.

41. Sacks FM, Pfeffer MA, Moye LA et al, The effect of pravastatin on coronary events after myocardial infarction in patients with average cholesterol levels, *N Engl J Med* 1996; **335:** 1001–9.

42. Long Term Intervention within Pravastatin In Ischaemic Disease (LIPID Study group), Prevention of cardiovascular events and death with pravastatin in patients with coronary heart disease and a broad range of initial cholesterol levels, *N Engl J Med* 1998; **339:** 1349–57.

43. Pyorala K, De Backer G, Graham I et al, on behalf of the Task Force, Prevention of coronary heart disease in clinical practice. Recommendations of the Task Force of the European Society of Cardiology, European Atherosclerosis Society and European Society of Hypertension, *Eur Heart J* 1998; **19:** 1434–503.

44. NHS Executive, SMAC Statement on Use of Statins. Executive Letter: EL (97)41 (Department of Health: Wetherby, West Yorkshire 1997).

45. Ad Hoc Subcommittee of the Liaison Committee of the WHO and the ISH, Effects of calcium antagonists on the risks of coronary heart disease, cancer and bleeding, *J Hum Hypertens* 1997; **11:** 331–42.

46. The Danish Study Group on Verapamil in Myocardial Infarction, Effect of verapamil on mortality and major events after acute myocardial infarction (the Danish Verapamil Infarction Trial II—DAVIT II), *Am J Cardiol* 1990; **66:** 779–85.

47. The Multicenter Diltiazem Postinfarction Trial Research Group, The effect of diltiazem on mortality and reinfarction after myocardial infarction, *N Engl J Med* 1988; **319:** 385–92.

48. The Cardiac Arrhythmia Suppression Trial

(CAST) Investigators, Preliminary report: effect of encainide and flecainide on mortality in a randomized trial of arrhythmia suppression after myocardial infarction, *N Engl J Med* 1989; **321**: 406–12.

49.   Teo KK, Yusuf S, Furberg CD, Effects of prophylactic antiarrhythmic drug therapy in acute myocardial infarction: an overview of results from randomised controlled trials, *JAMA* 1993; **270**: 1589–95.

50.   Waldo AL, Camm AJ, de Ruyter H et al, Effect of d-sotalol on mortality in patients with left ventricular dysfunction after recent and remote myocardial infarction, *Lancet* 1996; **348**: 7–12.

51.   Cairns JA, Connolly SJ, Roberts R, Gent M, Randomised trial of outcome after myocardial infarction in patients with frequent or repetitive ventricular premature depolarisations: CAMIAT, *Lancet* 1997; **349**: 675–82.

52.   Julian DG, Camm AJ, Frangin G et al, Randomised trial of effect of amiodarone on mortality in patients with left ventricular dysfunction after recent myocardial infarction: EMIAT, *Lancet* 1997; **349**: 667–74.

53.   Stampfer MJ, Colditz GA, Estrogen replacement therapy and coronary heart disease: a quantitative assessment of the epidemiologic evidence, *Preventive Med* 1991; **20**: 47–9.

54.   Diaz MN, Frei B, Vita JA, Keaney JF, Antioxidants and atherosclerotic heart disease, *N Engl J Med* 1997; **337**(6): 408–16.

55.   Sen S, Neuss H, Berg G et al, Beneficial effects of nicorandil in acute myocardial infarction: a placebo-controlled, double-blind pilot safety study, *Br J Cardiol* 1998; **5**: 208–20.

56.   Mendall MA, Inflammatory responses and coronary heart disease, *Br Med J* 1998; **316**: 953–4.

Index